Walking with God Through Cancer

WAYNE HASTINGS

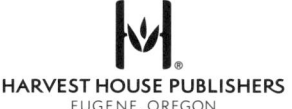

HARVEST HOUSE PUBLISHERS
EUGENE, OREGON

Scripture versions used can be found at the back of the book.

Cover design by Kyler Dougherty

Cover images © georgeclerk, Pobytov / Getty Images

Interior design by KUHN Design Group

For bulk, special sales, or ministry purchases, please call 1-800-547-8979. Email: CustomerService@hhpbooks.com

This logo is a federally registered trademark of the Hawkins Children's LLC. Harvest House Publishers, Inc., is the exclusive licensee of this trademark.

Walking with God Through Cancer
Copyright © 2025 by Wayne Hastings
Published by Harvest House Publishers
Eugene, Oregon 97408
www.harvesthousepublishers.com

ISBN 978-0-7369-9162-9 (Hardcover)
ISBN 978-0-7369-9163-6 (eBook)
Library of Congress Control Number: 2024952802

No part of this book may be used or reproduced in any manner for the purpose of training artificial intelligence technologies or systems.

All rights reserved. No part of this publication may be reproduced, stored in a retrieval system, or transmitted in any form or by any means—electronic, mechanical, digital, photocopy, recording, or any other—except for brief quotations in printed reviews, without the prior permission of the publisher.

Printed in China

25 26 27 28 29 30 31 32 33 / RDS / 10 9 8 7 6 5 4 3 2 1

*To those who need a sanctuary of hope,
a place of refuge in God's sustaining presence,
where comfort is found in the
unwavering promises of His Word,
and grace is abundantly given to navigate
your path with the light of faith.*

Table of Contents

Introduction 9

Part One: Discovering the Anchor of Grace

Day 1: Grace Through Faith 17

Day 2: Echoes of Grace 23

Day 3: Saved by Grace 27

Day 4: Life Changes Quickly 31

Day 5: Anchored by Grace 35

Part Two: Seasons of Change

Day 6: Navigating the Unknown 41

Day 7: Life's Side Effects 45

Day 8: Balancing Act 49

Day 9: Anchoring Hope 53

Day 10: Undertaking the Uncertainties of the Middle Ground 57

Part Three: Seeing Strength in Vulnerability

Day 11: Embracing Divine Vulnerability 63

Day 12: Breaking the Chains of Emotional Restraint 67

Day 13: Learning from a King 71
Day 14: Finding Hope Through Lament 75
Day 15: Flourishing in Vulnerability 79

Part Four: Embracing Moments of Joy

Day 16: Harmonizing Hope 85
Day 17: Embracing Joyful Gratitude 89
Day 18: Finding Shalom in the Stillness 93
Day 19: Two of Us. 97
Day 20: Finding Joy Despite All That's Bad 101

Part Five: Finding Purpose in the Journey

Day 21: Finding Purpose Through Difficulty 107
Day 22: Trusting God's Plan 111
Day 23: The Refining Fire 115
Day 24: The Good Shepherd 119
Day 25: Letting Your Light Shine 123

Part Six: Celebrating Small Victories

Day 26: Keep Going. 129
Day 27: Resetting Expectations 133
Day 28: From Grumbling to Gratitude 137
Day 29: Embracing Failures and Small Victories. . . 141
Day 30: Persistence and Small Wins 147

Part Seven: Trusting in God's Timing

Day 31: A Time for Patience 153

Day 32: Faith Is Waiting for God's Timing Without Knowing "When" 157

Day 33: Strength from Enduring Patience 161

Day 34: God's Timing and Patient Endurance 165

Day 35: Trusting in God's Timing 169

Part Eight: Welcoming Endurance and Hope

Day 36: Beyond the Thorn 175

Day 37: Choosing Hope When Everything Looks Hopeless 179

Day 38: The Power of Hope in God's Plan 183

Day 39: Embracing Hope over Negativity 187

Day 40: God's Anchor of Hope 191

Closing Thoughts: *Moving Forward* 195

Afterword 199

Notes 203

Introduction

Warm greetings to each of you embarking on this journey through the pages of *Walking with God Through Cancer: A 40-Day Devotional*. I welcome you to this devotional sanctuary with a heart filled with hope, faith, and a deep desire to extend grace.

The title, *Walking with God Through Cancer: A 40-Day Devotional*, encapsulates what I wish to share with you: what we discover when we walk daily with God, particularly through the tumultuous cancer journey. As someone intimately acquainted with the challenges of stage 4 cancer and second cancer, I extend my hand to you, fellow traveler, with the assurance that God's grace is not a distant concept but rather a tangible, transformative force that can carry us through life's roughest seas. This devotional is not just a collection of words, but a labor of love, faith, and vulnerability. It is an invitation to walk together, to find comfort in shared reflections, and to discover the threads of God's grace, love, presence, comfort, and peace woven through each of our stories.

Before we dive into the heart of these reflections, allow me to share a glimpse of my journey, an ongoing testament to His sustaining grace. In the summer of 2019, my life took an unexpected turn when I received a stage 4 cancer diagnosis. Amid the initial shock and the following whirlwind of emotions, I grappled with fear, uncertainty, and a profound sense of vulnerability. But in this storm, I heard God's fresh whispers of grace.

Then, in 2024, my oncologist told me I had B-cell lymphoma. This means I'm now, today, fighting two different cancers with two different types of treatment. But again, despite my fears, I have heard God's voice. God has demonstrated His grace to me in unexpected moments—during sleepless nights, through the unwavering support of loved ones, and in the courage He's given me to face each day with renewed hope. The more I studied the Bible and prayed, the more apparent it became that grace isn't the absence of obstacles on the path, but the sturdy walking stick that steadies me within its tumult. This devotional is an offering from these sacred, personal encounters with God's open arms of love, grace, and peace.

As you turn these pages, envision them as a haven where faith meets the reality of the cancer journey. Each reflection is a stepping stone, a gentle guide beckoning you to find grace in your storm. I cannot offer easy answers or quick fixes, but I can accompany you on the path of discovery and illuminate the way with the light of faith and resilience.

STRUCTURE OF THE DEVOTIONAL

The devotional is a pilgrimage—a journey of 40 reflections, each pertaining to the unique challenges, questions, and emotions accompanying the cancer journey. The path is not linear but a weaving narrative, mirroring the ebb and flow of life with cancer.

Days 1–5: Discovering the Anchor of Grace

Our voyage begins with exploring the anchor that grounds us—God's grace. Discover how His grace stabilizes us in the face of uncertainty and fear.

Days 6–10: Seasons of Change

The journey unfolds with reflections on navigating the unknown waters of diagnosis, treatment, and the myriad emotions that arise. Find encouragement in the assurance that you are not alone.

Days 11–15: Seeing Strength in Vulnerability

Vulnerability is not a weakness, but a source of strength. Explore how vulnerability opens the door to healing and a more fulfilling connection with the Lord.

Days 16–20: Embracing Moments of Joy

Within the storm, pockets of joy are waiting to be embraced. Delve into reflections that invite you to savor and celebrate moments of grace-filled joy.

Days 21–25: Finding Purpose in the Journey

Explore the profound question of purpose during illness. Uncover how this journey, despite its challenges, holds the potential for God's plans and purposes to be realized.

Days 26–30: Celebrating Small Victories

Focus on acknowledging and celebrating even the smallest triumphs. Seeking out others' inspirational stories of overcoming challenges can enable the recognition of your own victories.

Day 31–35: Trusting in God's Timing

Reflect on the significance of patience, trusting in God's timing and finding hope amid waiting as you lean on God's promises of renewed strength.

Day 36–40: Welcoming Endurance and Hope

Be encouraged to build character and hope through the cancer journey with reflections on the importance of hope as we strive to navigate the complex nature of this disease.

Closing Thoughts: Moving Forward

Be reminded and heartened through a summary of key lessons and insights gained from our time together.

As you embark on this journey, remember that you are not merely a reader; you are a fellow pilgrim. May these reflections be a balm to your soul, a source of inspiration, and a testament to the enduring grace accompanying you on your unique path.

As you read these pages, I ask you to commit to journaling as part of your daily devotional time. Keeping track of your thoughts will help you pour out your heart to the Lord and hear from Him. This exercise will enable you to revisit and review God's plan, purpose, and presence in your life, even amid chaos and uncertainty.

When the storms of life overwhelm, we may join with the words of the psalmist: "Let me take refuge under the shelter of your wings" (Psalm 61:4 ESV). May this devotional be a sanctuary, a refuge, as you navigate the path that's before you.

With love, grace, and unwavering hope,
Wayne Hastings

PART ONE

Discovering the Anchor of Grace

Let us come boldly to the throne of our gracious God. There we will receive his mercy, and we will find grace to help us when we need it most.

HEBREWS 4:16 NLT

DAY 1

Grace Through Faith

The word *grace* is beautiful. It's an expression of God's character and His interaction with us. The Hebrew Bible uses the word *chesed*, which means "grace, mercy, steadfast love, compassion."[1]

The New Testament holds several beautiful instances in which we witness God's *chesed*. In one noteworthy example in John 5, Jesus finds a man lying beside a healing pool, waiting for his chance for healing. The pool is called *Beit Chesed* in Hebrew, or *Bethzatha* in Aramaic, meaning "House of Loving-Kindness or Grace." Moved by compassion, Jesus heals the man instantly, demonstrating God's grace in action. This scene is a powerful reminder of God's limitless love and mercy toward us.

Later in the book of John, we find another instance of Jesus's kindness and compassion. In John 21, the disciples return to their old fishing profession, perhaps out of perplexity and anxiety over what had happened just a few days before. However, despite their efforts, they catch no fish. (Interestingly, the Hebrew word for fish is *dag*, which shares the same root as the Hebrew word for fear and anxiety.) This illustration reminds us that our efforts may result in empty nets when we operate from a place of fear. Jesus stands on the shore, but the disciples do not recognize Him:

> Then Jesus said to them, "Children, have you any food?" They answered Him, "No." And He said to them, "Cast the net on the right side of the boat, and you will find some." So, they cast, and now they were not able to draw it in because of the multitude of fish (John 21:5-6).

In Jewish thought, the left side is the side of severity and strict judgment. We can learn from this interaction that our nets will be empty when we live in a place of criticism and severity. But conversely in Judaism, the right side is the side of *chesed*, meaning God's lovingkindness, benevolence, and covenantal love. Nets fortified with love and *chesed*, God's grace, are abundantly supplied and enduring.

These two stories have relevance for those of us who are struggling with cancer or know someone who is. First, the man lying at the pool was just waiting for the next miracle. The man wanted Jesus to see things *his* way. Instead, Jesus told him to get up and walk, then told him to move on and live his life. Today, we face significant challenges as we endure this disease, but are we ready to accept God's *chesed*? Sure, choosing to rely on His power can be difficult; but God's presence, loving-kindness, and grace must be our focus. We may stumble, but we must keep our eyes on His *chesed* for us.

The disciples were living out of fear and anxiety—the left side of the boat. Jesus turned their focus to the right side—the side of His grace and full nets. This helps us understand that despite this disease, we can live with abundance because of God's grace. He loves us and wants our best. We can't outrun His grace. It transforms us from self-centered people into God-focused followers.

A CLOSING THOUGHT

David wrote in Psalm 86:15, "But you, O Lord, are a God of compassion and mercy, slow to get angry and filled with unfailing love and faithfulness" (NLT). Pastor David Platt said while teaching on this psalm,

> Based on who God had revealed himself to be through his words, David had not given up hope.[2]

David, despite difficult circumstances, didn't give up hope. Why? He believed in and clung to God's grace and loving-kindness.

REFLECTION

Take a moment and read Psalm 86, focusing mainly on verses 10-16.

- Under challenging circumstances, where did David turn?
- How would you describe David's attitude toward God's grace (*chesed*)?
- How would you describe your feelings about God's grace?
- Have you chosen to receive His grace to help you navigate the many challenges of this disease?

- How has any assistance you've received helped you to feel God's grace?

Now read Exodus 34:6-7. In your journal, make a list of the 13 qualities of God's mercy.

- What do these qualities tell you about God?
- How can these qualities help you better understand who God is and relate to His posture of grace and kindness?

DAY 2

Echoes of Grace

Every year in the quiet glow of post-Thanksgiving days, a cherished tradition unfolds in our home. My wife, Pam, transforms our house into a Christmas wonderland that flows from her heart full of holiday spirit. Once, when the laughter of our young children echoed through the walls, we had a different special tradition. Each year, Pam carefully chose and purchased ornaments for each of our children. Over the years, as every tiny capsule of meaning adorned the tree, it became a veritable scrapbook filled with precious memories of Christmases past.

Now our children are building their own stories, and the ornaments of their youth adorn their own trees. The tree in our home looks very different at Christmastime, but it remains an album of remembrance. It cradles keepsakes from our journey together, with some red ornaments dating back to our first Christmas as a married couple. Our tree has become a beautiful symbol of the importance of remembering.

Our dear friend Rabbi Jason Sobel, a Messianic rabbi, often emphasizes the importance of remembrance. He draws our attention to Jewish tradition, in which biblical holidays revolve around remembering. Two examples include Passover, in which the Jewish people recall the miraculous liberation from enslavement, and Purim, which urges remembrance of Queen Esther's courageous stand against the impending annihilation of the Jews and her acceptance of the challenge to step into history "for such a time as this" (Esther 4:14).

This year, as Pam hung each ornament delicately, I couldn't help but draw parallels. Like the Jewish holidays, our Christmas tree is a canvas for remembrance of all God has done in our lives. More than the shiny baubles and twinkling lights, the tree is a testimony to the big and small blessings, the triumphs, and the challenges overcome with the Lord's assistance, time and again.

We need to remember. Remember the laughter, the tears, the victories, and the lessons. Remembering the faithfulness of God is important amid every twist and turn of our journey.

As we navigate cancer's challenges and its related treatments, recollecting the times when God's presence and grace have been a tangible force in our lives, guiding us through trials and triumphs, can be helpful. These memories testify to His faithfulness and reassure us that the God who walked with us then is the same God walking with us now.

Every encounter with God shows us His unmatched grace. Whether He is calmly reassuring us during a sleepless night or providing overwhelming peace in the face of uncertainty, these moments carry us through the side effects and the persistent shadow of cancer.

During today's challenges, our memories remind us that the God who calmed our fears, provided strength in weakness, and revealed light in times of darkness is present with us right now. We draw strength from the well of past promises kept, whose waters flow unfailingly into the current challenges.

For anyone going through cancer, I invite you to remember the times when you felt God's presence flowing in and through your life. By doing so, you may be able to immerse yourself in the moments of grace from God, who will be with you in deep waters. I hope the memory of His faithfulness and love will spark hope and serve as a guiding light as you navigate each difficult stage of cancer.

A CLOSING THOUGHT

As we journey forward, let us embrace the truth that the God who has been our refuge, strength, and ever-present help in times past is the same God leading us triumphantly through the challenges of today. This idea is so beautifully expressed in the book *Exalting Jesus in Psalms 51–100*:

> God wants us to be gripped by the reality
> and emotion of what He's done for us.[1]

REFLECTION

Read Exodus 2:24-25 and Psalm 105:8. God heard the groanings of an enslaved people. Then, importantly, He remembered His covenantal promise to Abraham to prosper his descendants.

- In what ways is it important to know a God who remembers His promises?

- As you reflect upon God, do you remember His promises to you?

- In your journal, list some ways you can focus on God's promises on the days when things are challenging.

DAY 3

Saved by Grace

Isn't it interesting that upon meeting someone for the first time, we usually ask, "What do you do?" The question seems innocuous, but when we ask it, we are thinking about productivity and activity rather than the person. We live in a performance-oriented culture, and *doing* is at the forefront of our thinking. We celebrate pulling ourselves up by our bootstraps. We *do* so we can be promoted, get that raise, and deliver what others expect from us.

But for some of us, without warning, cancer enters our lives. We don't feel well. We are under treatments prescribed by others. Suddenly, there's not much we can *do*. We have no bootstraps to pull on. We find ourselves in a new community, under a doctor's care, and nothing we can *do* will change test results or outcomes. We can be smart—eat well, trust and be kind to our clinical team, and take our meds. But trying to do something on our own takes a back seat.

God's grace helps us transition from *doing* to *being*, by allowing us to rest in His loving care. God's grace is His unmerited favor. There is nothing we can do to earn it. He gives it freely as we trust Him with our circumstances.

Grace saves us spiritually, and His loving and long-suffering grace sustains us as we walk through cancer with Him. His grace is amazing. His grace is marvelous. And His grace leaves room for us to *do* things.

We can pray (Philippians 4:6). Prayer is the bridge to His peace because we cast our cares upon Him through it. Prayer joins us with God. We can't pray but then take our requests back and try to solve things independently. Prayer is also critical to spiritually nurturing God's promises in our lives. Prayer and God's Word keep His promises alive within our hearts and minds.

Our petitions should be as specific as possible. It is not enough to ask God to bless our family, faith community, nation, or even ourselves. We must pray for particular needs if we are to be effective prayers.

According to 1 Peter 5:7-8, we can cast our cares upon Him. Though only verse 7 tells us to pray, the verse that follows is connected. Peter tells us to cast our cares on God, be self-controlled, and not let anxiety take hold. But if we don't cast our cares upon a loving God, Peter warns us, the devil is prowling around like a roaring lion to devour us—bringing worry, anxiety, struggle, frustration, and strife into our lives. Your bright ideas, your efforts to change things in your own power, change nothing for the better and only invite stress.

Worrying doesn't solve problems. The stress of worrying weakens our already fragile internal systems. We are not smart enough to work ourselves out of our circumstances, so fearfully searching for answers is fruitless. The enemy would like to make us anxious about this disease—but God will defeat those anxieties. When we rest and cast our cares on God, He goes to work.

When you cast cares on Him, say, "God, I believe You are working on my challenges and circumstances." After that, you can wait for His work with patience and a good attitude (Psalm 46:10). Regarding Psalm 46:10, Charles Spurgeon said,

> Sit down and wait in patience, ye believers! Acknowledge that Jehovah is God, ye who feel the terrors of His wrath! Adore Him, and Him only, ye who partake in the protections of His grace.[1]

While dealing with cancer, we can sit and wait patiently for His purpose and His plan. We can choose stillness by dwelling in the protection of His saving grace.

A CLOSING THOUGHT

Sometimes we strive to *do* when we merely need to pray, rest in the Lord, and have an attitude of patience and kindness.

REFLECTION

Read Philippians 4:6. Take a few moments and go directly to God with praise, prayer, and thanksgiving. In your prayer, praise Him for what He will do and be anxious for nothing. During this time with God, let the great peace of God enter your heart.

Read 1 Peter 5:7-8.

- What does it mean to cast your cares upon God?
- List the cares you need to cast upon the Lord in your journal. Then, mentally cast them upon Him and rest in His peace.

DAY 4

Life Changes Quickly

To turn on a dime is to "suddenly change completely or do something completely different from what [you] were doing before." The idea behind this phrase is of "being able to change direction quickly and easily in a very small space, as if your foot were on a coin."[1]

Amid the treatment for my stage 4 prostate cancer, I suddenly found myself turning on a dime.

My oncologist was straightforward but optimistic when he told me the chemotherapy I'd received hadn't erased all the metastasized cells. He recommended an infusion-type radiation that would target and attack only those errant cells. I received one treatment, and in a follow-up appointment, my blood panel numbers were strange. I needed a blood transfusion and checked into the hospital. I spent four days there, and over the course of those four days, the outstanding medical staff determined I had a second cancer: B-cell lymphoma.

Once home, I was weak and needed more transfusions. A few days after my first chemotherapy treatment for lymphoma, I passed out, and EMS took me to the hospital again. It took 12 days for my blood count to normalize enough for the doctors to release me.

Over just a few weeks, my life and the lives of my family members had turned on a dime.

While the days are extremely challenging, God is faithful and gracious. We have experienced daily blessings. Yes, we've had emotional moments, challenges, weariness, and separation from each other, but God's mercy and grace have carried us through.

Reflecting again on Psalm 46, I notice a reminder that God is our refuge and strength. When things turn on a dime, we have a God whose strength and grace never wane. We have a God who is our refuge. The definition of the Hebrew word for refuge invokes a quiet place to go for protection. We have a God whose strength sustains and protects us when things crumble.

Psalm 46:10 reminds us, "Be still, and know that I am God." Bible teacher and author James Montgomery Boice commented,

> [Verse 10] means rather, "Lay down your arms. Surrender and acknowledge that I am the one and only victorious God." Of course,

the time to do this is now, while a desirable peace can be yours through the work of Jesus on the cross.[2]

When our lives are so quickly altered, we must surrender and acknowledge that God has a purpose and a plan for us. He is sovereign. He knows the beginning from the end.

Surrendering doesn't mean giving up. We can fervently pray. We can take responsibility for what our doctors have prescribed. We can be grateful and caring and have a positive attitude toward our caregivers and the people we meet. We can drop seeds so people see our faith in action as we work through the challenges of a rapidly changing personal landscape.

God sustains. When the paths of our lives suddenly veer off into uncharted territories, He is our strength and refuge. We can be still and know that He is God. We can rest in His arms, knowing He has things under control. We can be still and relax.

A CLOSING THOUGHT

On the day he was passing away, John Wesley's voice had almost completely faded, making him difficult to understand. Yet, with his remaining strength, Wesley suddenly cried out, "The best of all is, God is with us." Then, raising his hand triumphantly, he repeated with a powerful impact, "The best of all is, God is with us."[3] Do you feel God's presence and strength when your life changes quickly?

REFLECTION

Read Deuteronomy 31:8. Here, we find Moses encouraging Joshua for his upcoming assignment to become the new leader of the children of Israel.

- In what ways has God encouraged you? How does His encouragement help you be still when life changes rapidly?

Read Psalm 4:8. Ask the Lord to show you how to shut out the noise of changing circumstances and, through prayer and Scripture, feel only His peace, find His refuge, and hear His voice.

DAY 5

Anchored by Grace

Every Sunday, our church prays for people with various needs. Unfortunately, cancer is often one of those prayed-for requests. The disease has no boundaries. It reaches every demographic, gender, and race. When you're diagnosed with cancer, the ground beneath you seems to give way. Fear, uncertainty, and sorrow race through your mind. But in these unsettled moments, God's grace is our steadfast anchor. His grace not only sustains us, but also transforms our lives into testimonies of faith and resilience.

God freely gives His grace. It is a gift we cannot earn. His grace reminds us we are never alone, even in the face of a cruel disease. Paul, in his New Testament letter to the Corinthians, shared a profound truth about grace: "My grace is sufficient for you, for my power is made perfect in weakness" (2 Corinthians 12:9 NIV). In our weakest moments, God's grace becomes our strength.

Grace is a lifeline that steadies us when we feel overwhelmed by the reality of cancer.

Cancer brings a whirlwind of emotions and challenges. Physical pain, emotional distress, and spiritual questioning can accompany the diagnosis and treatment. In our moments of vulnerability, God's grace becomes most evident. Grace is not just a comforting word; it is an active force that works in our lives. It brings peace that surpasses understanding (Philippians 4:7) and hope that does not disappoint (Romans 5:5).

As we walk through cancer, each day presents unique challenges; but God's grace provides us the strength to face them. Isaiah 40:31 assures us, "Those who wait on the Lord shall renew their strength; they shall mount up with wings like eagles, they shall run and not be weary, they shall walk and not faint." This strength is a testament to God's sustaining power, enabling us to endure treatments, cope with side effects, and maintain hope.

The journey through cancer is fraught with uncertainties. Yet God's grace provides a peace that guards our hearts and minds. Jesus said, "Peace I leave with you; my peace I give you. I do not give to you as the world gives. Do not let your hearts be troubled and do not be afraid" (John 14:27 NIV). This peace reassures us that

God is sovereign. He holds our future, no matter how uncertain and complicated a situation seems.

As we experience God's grace alongside our diagnoses, our lives become testimonies of His faithfulness. God transforms our trials into stories of hope and resilience. We learn to trust in God more deeply, finding that His grace is sufficient.

Cancer may change many aspects of our lives, but it cannot diminish the power of God's grace. His grace anchors us, giving us the strength to persevere, the comfort to endure, and the peace to face each day with hope. Through God's grace, we can stand firm.

A CLOSING THOUGHT

For a cancer patient, trusting in God's unfailing gift of grace means finding peace and strength amid uncertainty and fear. We can be assured that God's love and grace are constant, even when we face the trials of illness. God's grace provides comfort as we remember that He is present in every moment, offering us peace that surpasses understanding. Trusting God enables the patient to surrender their anxieties to Him—to rest in the belief that His plans are ultimately good, even when they are difficult to understand.

REFLECTION

This devotion closes this section. Reflect on some of the Bible verses you have read in today's devotion. I encourage you to reread them slowly and thoughtfully. As you reread them, consider all the times you've experienced God's grace and write about them in your journal. Remembering the times when His grace kept you and anchored you will give you strength for tomorrow.

PART TWO

Seasons of Change

*The L*ORD *himself goes before you and will be with you; he will never leave you nor forsake you. Do not be afraid; do not be discouraged.*

DEUTERONOMY 31:8 NIV

DAY 6

Navigating the Unknown

One of the first songs I learned to play on my guitar was "Turn! Turn! Turn!" I first heard Pete Seeger's version; then, in 1965, I fell in love with Roger McGuinn and the Byrds' version of the iconic song.

Seeger wrote the song in 1959 as he was "just leafing through" the Bible. According to music writer Steve Turner, "So moved was [Seeger] by the ancient poetry that he began creating a melody to which the words could be sung."[1] The Byrds' version topped the charts in 1965 and remains a mainstay of McGuinn's live performances.

The song (with a few minor tweaks from Seeger) comes from King Solomon's writing in Ecclesiastes. The wise king wrote in Ecclesiastes 3:1-8 that there is a time and season for everything under heaven, including birth, death, planting, harvesting, mourning, dancing, and peace. The ancient words highlight the balance and order in life's events.

Solomon's poignant words remind us that life unfolds in seasons, each with its appointed time. From moments of birth to moments of loss, from times of joy to times of sorrow, every experience has its place in God's plan. As Pastor Charles Swindoll aptly said, "There is an appointed time for everything."[2]

Embracing change isn't always easy. We all progress through various seasons of life, but we often don't move willingly. We may feel the cold weather coming, but we resist the change of seasons. We may struggle to let go of the pleasantly familiar. We may enjoy fall and hate winter, but the fated transition has an appointed time.

Facing change as a caregiver or cancer patient—whether you're adapting to new treatments or navigating shifts in health conditions—is such a struggle. Coping with the challenges and navigating the transitions with grace, resilience, and peace requires biblical wisdom and practical insight.

We've learned we must trust God's sovereignty. Remember King Solomon's words: Each season has an appointed time. God is sovereign and faithful, and He is the Director of all seasons of life.

During our current seasons of change, Pam and I have had to stop thinking about what we're facing and turn to prayer as a source of comfort and strength. We are constantly learning to surrender our fears and anxieties about changes and seek to trust God (Philippians 4:6-7).

We've also discovered that finding truth is better than trusting emotions and our human thought processes. We often need to take the initiative to educate ourselves about conditions and treatments. Even more, we find and cling to the truth in Scripture.

You can embrace other biblical and practical ideas that will help you through seasons of change. We all can find strength, resilience, and peace amid the uncertainties. Remember that you are not alone; God is with you every step of the way, guiding you through the changes and leading you toward healing and wholeness.

A CLOSING THOUGHT

To quote Pastor Warren Wiersbe,

> If we cooperate with God's timing, life will not be meaningless. Everything will be "beautiful in his time" [Ecclesiastes 3:11], even the most difficult experiences of life.[3]

REFLECTION

Read Joshua 1:9, where we find Joshua facing an enormous task.

- How do God's words to Joshua prepare him for the changes ahead?

- In what ways can embracing change strengthen your trust in God?

- How can focusing on God's promises provide comfort during uncertain times?

DAY 7

Life's Side Effects

Most of the time, cancer involves navigating the unknown. The disease has both overt and covert qualities, and it can move and operate in the dark. Side effects are one of those unknowns. Unfortunately and inevitably, cancer treatments—from medications to chemotherapy to radiation—make their presence felt. While undergoing several treatments, as I've anticipated and endured drug-related side effects, I can't help but think of the disclaimers rattled off in those pharmaceutical commercials, the ones where the rapid-fire narration lists potential consequences at breakneck speed.

Throughout several treatments, I experienced the brunt of side effects—something my nurses and the oncologist's office have often observed their patients enduring. As I navigated the discomfort and pain, I discovered that the key is learning to roll with the punches and keep the bigger picture in focus.

Contemplating the concept of side effects led me to reflect on other, non-drug-related consequences that arise in our everyday lives. Decisions, akin to medications, can yield both positive and negative effects. Take antihistamines, for instance. They are great for clearing congestion, but they potentially induce drowsiness too. Just so, we face life choices every day, each one with its accompanying consequences. Speeding on the highway may lead to a hefty traffic ticket or even incarceration, if a state trooper is involved. Likewise, King David faced dire consequences for staying home from battle and succumbing to temptation when he observed Bathsheba. Contrastingly, Joseph—despite doing the right thing by resisting Potiphar's wife—found himself in prison but eventually rose to prominence as the second in command of Egypt. Choices, much like medications, have consequences.

My life, too, has been marked by decisions that ushered in both positive and detrimental outcomes. Yet one decision I made long ago stands out, having led to only positive side effects: In 1979, I embraced Jesus the Messiah as my personal Lord and Savior. In the face of life's challenges, even cancer, His presence, peace, guidance, wisdom, and grace have been my unwavering companions. I cherish His Word, His Spirit, His promises, and the assurance that He listens to every prayer. "He only is my rock and my salvation; He is my defense; I shall not be greatly moved" (Psalm 62:2).

We all make decisions with ensuing side effects, but trust me: The decision to welcome Jesus into your life every minute of every day is the best decision you can make…with no harmful effects.

A CLOSING THOUGHT

Pastor Charles Stanley wrote,

> My observation has been that the more a person focuses on himself, the less he is able to keep his life in order. On the other hand, the more an individual focuses on Christ, the easier it becomes to allow Him to control every area of life.[1]

REFLECTION

Take a moment to read John 3:16, a familiar passage to many. Study the words and phrases the apostle John used to describe the invitation to receive Jesus:

- God so loved the world
- that He gave

- His only begotten Son,
- that whoever believes in Him
- should not perish but have everlasting life.

In your journal, describe each line in your own words and what it means to you. How do these phrases and words help you cope with life's side effects?

DAY 8

Balancing Act

Battling cancer has been made bearable by firmly holding God's hand and having an incredible caregiver in my beloved wife, Pam. She has been a spiritual and emotional rock, praying, encouraging, sympathizing, and enduring my varying moods and reactions to the disease and chemotherapy's side effects. She advises, hugs, and listens as we both walk the path of the unknown.

Amid their own challenges, patients need to recognize the needs of caregivers—emotional, physical, relational, and spiritual. How do our caregivers walk the tightrope to meet both their needs and ours? Such a delicate balance requires attention and care.

In the Old Testament book of Ruth, we find a poignant and inspiring story of a grief-stricken widow, Naomi, and her devoted daughter-in-law, Ruth. After the death of Naomi's husband and the premature demise of her own husband, Ruth chooses to stay with Naomi, proclaiming, "Wherever you go, I will go; and wherever you lodge, I will lodge; your people shall be my people, and your God, my God" (Ruth 1:16). Ruth's declaration is a beautiful portrayal of a caregiver offering unwavering support to someone in pain, as she willingly turns from the familiar to the unknown.

Indeed, tending to a caregiver's and a patient's emotional, spiritual, and physical needs is crucial. Several biblical principles can help us find balance by taking the reassuring hand of God.

Philippians 2:3-4 reminds us to

> Do nothing out of selfish ambition or vain conceit. Rather, in humility value others above yourselves, not looking to your own interests but each of you to the interests of the others (NIV).

Ruth displayed a selfless approach by prioritizing her mother-in-law during their time of grief. As patients, we need to recognize when our caregivers have needs too.

In Galatians 6:2, the apostle Paul wrote, "Share each other's burdens, and in this way obey the law of Christ" (NLT). Here we find the importance of mutual support and shared burdens. British Anglican priest and theologian John Stott reminds us

> Notice the assumption which lies behind this command, namely that we **all have burdens** and that **God does not mean us to carry them alone**. Of course **we** can cast **all** our **burdens** on Christ, but one of the ways he bears our **burdens** is through human friendship. To be a **burden** bearer is a great ministry[1] (emphasis mine).

First Corinthians 16:14 tells us, "Let all that you do be done in love" (ESV). This verse encourages a loving and supportive approach between caregiver and patient, each considering the other's emotional and spiritual well-being. It is also important to acknowledge that you're both probably finding yourselves in uncharted territory.

Practically, the caregiver and patient must encourage open and honest communication, which will foster an environment where both caregiver and patient can express their needs and concerns.

Caregivers should prioritize self-care activities, such as regular breaks, exercise, and moments of relaxation. These activities ensure they maintain their own physical and emotional well-being. Pam loves to garden and paint. These activities allow her to be creative, give her time to relax, and provide much-needed breaks from the rigors of giving care.

A CLOSING THOUGHT

As we navigate the unknowns of cancer, balancing the needs of both caregiver and patient requires intention, effort, understanding, and a commitment to mutual well-being.

REFLECTION

The book of Ruth is a beautiful story of friendship, caregiving, and generosity. Read the book of Ruth and note in your journal how the primary players (Naomi, Ruth, and Boaz) care for each other. Note how God works through these ordinary people to bring kindness and caring as they venture into new, uncertain, and possibly fearful situations.

DAY 9

Anchoring Hope

When I was ten, my parents took me on a tour of a World War II battleship. It was impressive to walk through the many sections of the ship. The guns were huge, and I also remember the size of the anchor. Of course the anchor *had* to be massive to keep that large ship tethered while being buffeted by the sea's waves. The ocean is rarely calm; the anchor keeps the boat from floating away once it's moored. When the anchor is lowered to the seabed, the ship is secure.

Amid life's most turbulent and uncharted seas, finding an anchor becomes essential. For those navigating the uncertain journey of cancer, whether as patients or caregivers, this need for stability and hope is deeply felt. Hebrews 6:19 presents a powerful metaphor that speaks directly to this need: "We have this hope as an anchor for the soul, firm and secure" (NIV). When circumstances are unknown, this message of hope is not a spiritual platitude but a foundational truth that provides tangible comfort and guidance when we may have no clue what the future will bring. *The Message* Bible restates Hebrews 6:19 by describing the anchor of hope as "an unbreakable spiritual lifeline."

Theologian and pastor John Piper said,

> What anchors our soul is not our subjective confidence, but the sure objective reality that God has promised. This is our anchor.[1]

Keeping to this theme, British author and Bible teacher A.W. Pink wrote,

> In Scripture (e.g., Romans 8:25; Hebrews 6:18-19) hope signifies a firm expectation and confident anticipation of the things God has promised. As joy and peace increase "in believing" so too does hope.[2]

Hebrews 6:19 offers more than a symbol for hope; it provides a promise. In the context of faith, hope is not wishful thinking. It is a confident expectation based on the character and promises of God, the Creator of all things. Biblical hope serves as an anchor for cancer patients because it is "firm and secure," unwavering even in the face of uncertainty. This hope does not deny the reality of suffering but rather offers a steadfastness rooted in Someone greater than the situation at hand. This Someone is so powerful, nothing is too complex or complicated for Him (Jeremiah 32:17).

My understanding of an anchor of hope is finding peace in the present moment. To achieve this peace, Pam and I cherish each day as a gift. Even though the future may seem uncertain, finding quiet moments of joy and gratitude helps anchor us in the present and provides stability and grace during troubling times.

Searching for uplifting Scriptures and affirmations in the Bible can offer you strength and hope. God's Word is a soothing balm, providing solace during challenging times.

Consider the story of Job, who, despite immense suffering, remained anchored in his faith. Ponder, too, the many who found healing and comfort through their encounters with Jesus. Today, similar stories unfold in hospitals and homes worldwide, where the power of hope changes despair into resilience. These stories remind us that hope is available even when everything seems uncertain.

A CLOSING THOUGHT

For those who have been affected by cancer and the uncertainty that surrounds it, Hebrews 6:19 invites you to put your hope in the Lord. This hope doesn't guarantee an easy journey, but it provides grace, strength, peace, and a sense of security—a blessed assurance.

REFLECTION

Read Job 19:25-27, where Job expresses a deep yearning to see God even during his suffering.

- What does this passage teach you about maintaining a heavenly perspective while facing the unknown?

- How can focusing on the promise of eternal life with God provide comfort and strength in your current battle with cancer?

DAY 10

Undertaking the Uncertainties of the Middle Ground

The middle is an unsettling place to be. We can look backward and realize how far we've come, or we can look forward to see how far we must go. Or we can remain stuck in the middle, going neither forward nor backward.

At certain moments in life we will find ourselves caught in the throes of indecision, fear, or regret. We feel stuck at a crossroads with paths diverging in multiple directions. In such a place, the weight of choices hangs in the air, and the future seems uncertain. Like a baseball player caught between bases, hesitant to move forward or retreat, we can experience the middle as both a challenging and a reflective space. Once again, drawing inspiration from the wisdom found in the Bible, Ecclesiastes 3:1 reminds us: "There's an opportune time to do things, a right time for everything on the earth" (MSG). This timeless truth speaks to the ebb and flow of decisions in our lives, emphasizing the importance of discerning the right moment to embrace uncertainty with a heart attuned to the Lord's guidance.

In Exodus 14, we find the children of Israel stuck in the middle. The Red Sea blocked their path forward. The most formidable army in the ancient world raced behind them. Because of their fear, some of them wanted to return to being enslaved people. But Moses, their leader, told them, "Do not be afraid" (Exodus 14:13). Then the Lord spoke directly to Moses, saying: "Tell the children of Israel to go forward" (Exodus 14:15).

The children of Israel were wallowing in indecision; God told them to move ahead despite their uncertainty. They were in the middle, stuck in a place of not knowing. Isn't that like God? He often asks us to step out in faith before He steps in. Sometimes, we must be in over our heads before God provides the dry ground. When we're in the middle, we must be willing to take risks according to God's leading and be unmoved by our fears, doubts, and indecision. We have to step into the unknown and attempt the seemingly impossible with our God, who promises to be our strength (Psalm 28:7;

Philippians 4:13), give us wisdom (James 1:5), and be present with us through every hardship (1 Corinthians 10:13; 1 Peter 5:7).

God had a purpose for the crossroads He placed before the children of Israel. He wanted His people to choose to allow Him to lead them into a place of blessing. We can't let cancer keep us in the middle. If we risk going forward, we will experience all that God has for us.

In the cancer treatment experience, the unknown looms. However, let's not dwell on the uncertainties of the middle ground. Instead, let's embrace the path ahead with hope and determination, fortified by the assurance of God's presence. Like the children of Israel who walked through the Red Sea, we can also move forward confidently, knowing that God takes care of His own. Yes, we may face challenges, but with God's help, we can confront and overcome them, stepping into the future He has ordained for us.

A CLOSING THOUGHT

In the face of fear, let's draw inspiration from God's call to the children of Israel to "go forward." We can be confident that the journey ahead, though challenging, is guided by the Lord's hand, leading us toward healing and purpose.

REFLECTION

Read Nehemiah 4:1-6. Notice in verse six that the wall was "half its height." We typically are discouraged when we are halfway through something. In the middle, we can't easily see the beginning or the end.

In your journal, describe an experience when you felt stuck in the middle.

- How did it feel?
- How can God help you "go forward" when you're in the middle?

PART THREE

Seeing Strength in Vulnerability

Jesus wept.

JOHN 11:35

DAY 11

Embracing Divine Vulnerability

Our instincts often lead us to shield ourselves from physical or emotional harm. We fasten seat belts, don helmets, and wrap ourselves in protective armor against the uncertainties of our journey. Yet a subtler safeguard exists—one that not only protects us against physical harm, but also seeks to strengthen us emotionally.

Many of us pursue emotional invincibility to shield ourselves from hurt. We inadvertently build walls that stifle the genuine expression of our feelings. While offering a semblance of security, this self-preserving armor can inflict wounds as we suppress our honest emotions.

I often reflect on a pivotal point at which I found myself a few years ago. The outcome of a biopsy forced me to face the limits of invulnerability. The desire to be tough and stand firm in the face of challenging news collided with the reality of my inner anxiety. Tears readily flowed and mingled with the shared emotions of my wife. In that vulnerable moment, my façade of invincibility crumbled, and the assertive, logical person within me discovered strength—not in emotional protection, but in letting go and embracing vulnerability.

The Scriptures illuminate the paradoxical strength found in vulnerability. The apostle Paul, in his second letter to the Corinthians, wrote of uncovering God's strength in human weakness: "[God] said to me, 'My grace is sufficient for you, for my power is made perfect in weakness'" (2 Corinthians 12:9 NIV). This verse refers to Paul's ongoing battle, which he called his "thorn in the flesh." Bible commentator Dr. Colin Kruse wrote,

> Having been taught that Christ's power is made perfect in weakness, Paul is glad to boast of his *weaknesses*. This does not mean he enjoys weaknesses as such; what he delights in is the power of Christ that rests upon him in these weaknesses.[1]

Amid the tears shed and the emotions laid bare, I encountered a profound truth: that vulnerability is not a sign of weakness, but a conduit for the Lord's strength. In His grace, our Lord meets us in our moments of deepest need. During these times of intense openness, God can bring about transformation in our lives.

Society often perpetuates the myth that strength lies in invulnerability, behind an unyielding wall shielding us from the rawness of our emotions. However, I've discovered that the cancer pathway dismantles this illusion, inviting us to confront our vulnerability head on. Vulnerability is not a surrender, but a courageous willingness to stand open and unafraid, declaring, "I am here—fragile, yet resilient—firmly holding God's hand."

A CLOSING THOUGHT

Vulnerability becomes a precious connection—a place where we meet God's boundless grace. It is not a surrender to weakness but—as demonstrated by the apostle Paul—a courageous acknowledgment of our need for His support.

REFLECTION

Study Isaiah 43:2.

- In your own words, describe what it means to be vulnerable.

- Why is it dangerous for us to hide or cover up our feelings, especially when we are hurting emotionally?

- In those times when you have felt weak or vulnerable, describe the comfort you have received in knowing that the Lord is with you.

DAY 12

Breaking the Chains of Emotional Restraint

My father grew up during the Great Depression, in the heart of Kansas's dust bowl. His father suffered a severe head wound in World War I and had difficulty working full-time. Consequently, my father went to work at the tender age of eight, digging trenches for the railroad. Dad was a veteran of World War II and a successful businessman. He rarely showed any vulnerability. My father would laugh and display anger, but as I was growing up, he didn't cry or let my mother or me see his emotions. Not until much later in his life did I see him weep and let go of the façade of invulnerability.

The emotional restraints we impose on ourselves can become chains that hinder the free flow of God's grace and help. Like a locked door, these restraints prevent the warmth of His love from permeating every corner of our lives. King David beautifully captured the liberation found in vulnerability: "The LORD is near to those who have a broken heart, and saves such as have a contrite spirit" (Psalm 34:18). The Hebrew word translated as "contrite" is *dakka*: "an adjective meaning destruction, a crumbled substance or pulverized dust...by extension it means humble or contrite."[1]

Vulnerability becomes a healing balm for the soul. Pastor Warren Wiersbe pointed out that when you're free to be vulnerable, "God's eyes see your needs, God's ears hear your prayers, and God is near you when your heart is broken."[2]

As we work through our cancer ordeal, we must heed the call to vulnerability, recognizing that our emotional authenticity is not a liability but a channel for God's power. We discover a strength that surpasses our understanding in the space of vulnerability. This strength flows directly from the wellspring of God's grace and love.

May we, like the psalmist, declare with open hearts: "Create in me a clean heart, O God, and renew a steadfast [firm, stable, established[3]] spirit within me" (Psalm 51:10). In vulnerability, we find a flow of renewal from our Father and strength beyond measure.

As cancer patients, we are not defined by our vulnerabilities. The strength we summon in acknowledging and embracing our weakness defines us. Vulnerability becomes a wellspring of resilience—strength that empowers us to face treatment challenges, endure the uncertainties of prognosis, and find meaning in the storm. In our vulnerability, we open a space for the Lord to work wonders. There, He can transform our moments of emotional exposure into opportunities for His strength to shine.

In vulnerability, we uncover the paradoxical truth that strength flourishes in fragility. Like a flower breaking through a tiny crack in the sidewalk, our resilience—with God's help—emerges from the cracks of vulnerability.

A CLOSING THOUGHT

May we find the courage to embrace our vulnerability, knowing that in doing so, we unearth a well of God's strength to sustain us on this challenging journey.

REFLECTION

Read 2 Kings 22:19. King Josiah had a tender heart. In Hebrew, the word translated *tender* means humility of heart and strength before God.

- Why do you need a humble heart to be open and vulnerable to what you're experiencing?

- Why do you suppose many people think having a tender heart is wrong?

- How does a tender heart show strength before God?

DAY 13

Learning from a King

King David was many things. He was a shepherd, a warrior, a songwriter, and the founder of a royal dynasty that eventually birthed the Messiah, Jesus. As a teenager, David defeated Goliath; as a young man, David was pursued by King Saul, who wanted to kill him. David committed adultery, yet he was also a man after God's own heart (Acts 13:22). King David lived a triumphant yet sometimes troubled life. He also expressed deep emotions and unwavering trust in the Lord. Rabbi Menachem Posner wrote this about David:

> Throughout his life, David expressed his emotion through song and/or weeping. Even though he was a celebrated warrior, David was not ashamed to show his humanity. Like David, we must give expression to our feelings, never feeling too "manly" for a good cry.[1]

David expressed himself in many ways, and perhaps the most famous expressions are his writings in the book of Psalms. In Jewish culture, the psalms were worship music. They were meant to be sung. Their lyrics, like many songs today, are poetry expressing everything from complete trust in the Lord to feelings of joy, thanksgiving, sadness, lament, grief, despair, and hope. The writers didn't hold back. They wrote from a perspective of vulnerability.

David wrote Psalm 51 following his adulterous relationship with Bathsheba (2 Samuel 11:2-5) and the prophet Nathan's confrontation (2 Samuel 12).

> Have mercy upon me, O God,
> According to Your lovingkindness;
> According to the multitude of Your tender mercies,
> Blot out my transgressions.
> Wash me thoroughly from my iniquity,
> And cleanse me from my sin.
> For I acknowledge my transgressions,
> And my sin is always before me (Psalm 51:1-3).

David opened himself to the Lord. He asked for mercy. He admitted his sin. David confessed having trouble shaking his guilt. In verse eight, David revealed that God had "broken" his bones, yet he was also open enough to ask God to restore his joy.

David ended this psalm asking God to restore his joy (verse 12), deliver him from guilt (verse 14), and enable him to praise to God (verse 15). What a beautiful example of a person being open and vulnerable. Adopting his excellent example of openness can lead us to worship God and understand His mercy and grace. For those of us who are at some stage of cancer, we can learn from David how vulnerably acknowledging our anger, frustration, and pain will help us on this journey.

Exodus 34:6-7 shows us some qualities of God's mercy as God declares that He is "merciful and gracious, longsuffering, and abounding in goodness and truth, keeping mercy for thousands, forgiving iniquity and transgression and sin." It was this mercy David sought when he turned to God, seeking His mercy, prayerfully and powerfully crying out to Him.

At one point, I spent considerable time in the hospital. My immune system was compromised, and I was in virtual isolation. I was scared; yet when I cried out to God, sometimes only praying, *Help me, Jesus,* my attitude significantly changed. I didn't feel alone. I admitted I needed God's help.

Several of David's psalms vacillate between complete trust in God and intense emotional affliction. In his writing, David never holds back his feelings; but at the same time, he never loses sight of God's mercy and compassion.

A CLOSING THOUGHT

As we manage cancer, let's look at King David's example. He was a mighty warrior, a powerful king…and a man who was unafraid to admit his feelings. He truly understood the struggles of life and beautifully conveyed his heartfelt emotions through his psalms and prayers.

REFLECTION

Read and study both Psalms 31 and 51.

- How did David let God know how he felt?
- How did he demonstrate his trust in God?
- Can you recall a situation in which you felt like a "broken vessel," as described in Psalm 31:12? How did you seek God's help?
- How did being open with the Lord help you in challenging times?

DAY 14

Finding Hope Through Lament

ament is a seldom-used word. *Collins Dictionary* says:

> Someone's *lament* is an expression of their sadness, regret, or disappointment about something.[1]

I believe a lament is the cry of a heart reaching out to God in a way that conveys profound pain that defies any other form of expression. In these moments, God intimately understands our suffering. Through lament, we express our pain and glimpse God's heart—His profound empathy for our struggles and His unwavering love and grace.

Amid deep lament, experiencing hope can be difficult

for us. The physical and emotional pain we feel from this disease can obscure our view of God's promises. Yet it's essential to remember that God works through every situation, and lament is never fruitless. Think of a diamond, which must endure intense pressure to emerge beautiful and pure. Similarly, God is at work in our pain, refining us through the pressure of lament. In His refinement, we find hope.

We often find it easy to suppress our emotions, hiding them away like the squirrels in my backyard hoarding food. But we can't be afraid to embrace our lament. The Bible tells of many people who lamented openly. Through their honest cries, God worked and transformed their lives. When we allow ourselves to lament, we seize an opportunity to connect deeply with God, who opens a channel and goes to work in our lives. As David did in many psalms, we can come to grips with our emotions and cast them to our loving heavenly Father in the crucible of lament.

Remember the death of Lazarus (John 11)? When Jesus arrived and found Lazarus dead, He didn't immediately fix the situation, even though He had the power to do so. Instead, He took time to lament and weep with His friends and family. By lamenting, we follow Jesus's example, allowing God to work through our pain and lead us to His love, mercy, and compassion.

As we navigate the challenges of cancer, we can embrace moments of lament. We can cry out to God with our pain, knowing He hears and understands. Our tears can be signs that we trust God enough to bring our deepest sorrows before Him. In our laments, God is working, refining our spirits, and preparing us for the hope He has for us.

Lament is not a sign of weakness but a step toward healing. In our moments of vulnerability, God's strength is made perfect. We can allow ourselves to fully experience our pain and sorrow and trust that God is with us every step of the way. Through lament, we will find hope, and in that hope, we will uncover the strength to persevere through cancer's challenges.

A CLOSING THOUGHT

As we grapple with cancer, we can find solace in God's presence and hope in His promises. We can lament deeply, but also look forward with hope, knowing that God is at work.

REFLECTION

Psalms 42 and 43 are psalms of lament. They freely express the psalmist's inner thoughts and feelings.

- What does it mean to you to pour out your soul to God?

- How does studying these psalms help you open up to God and others about your feelings?

- The psalmist turns to God with his sorrow. Take time to journal your genuine feelings about your circumstances and your openness to God's leading and help.

DAY 15

Flourishing in Vulnerability

As we've discussed in previous devotions, we often perceive vulnerability as a weakness. We build walls around our hearts, trying to protect ourselves from emotions like hurt and disappointment. However, when it comes to our relationship with God, these walls can hinder the intimate connection He desires to have with us. When we tear down these barriers, we can find genuine spiritual growth and intimacy with God. As the psalmists and even Jesus model for us, we can bare our souls before Him.

Prayer and worship are powerful ways to connect with God. When we come before Him with open hearts, sharing our deepest fears, struggles, and desires, we invite His presence into our lives in a transformative way. Hebrews 4:15-16 reminds us of this truth:

> This High Priest of ours [Jesus] understands our weaknesses, for he faced all of the same testings we do, yet he did not sin. So let us come boldly to the throne of our gracious God. There we will receive his mercy, and we will find grace to help us when we need it most (NLT).

Jesus endured pain and suffering, yet He never hesitated to approach God's throne boldly. Church of Scotland minister and Bible commentator William Barclay wrote,

> When we have a sad and sorry tale to tell, when life has drenched us with tears, we do not go to a God who is incapable of understanding what has happened; we go to a God who has been there.[1]

When we are vulnerable with God, we create space for His presence to dwell more deeply within us. Vulnerability in prayer means being honest about our doubts, confessing our sins, and expressing our deepest longings. In worship, it means praising Him even when we don't feel like it, trusting His goodness amid our pain and uncertainties.

As we pray and worship, we acknowledge our dependence on Him. This openness expands our relationship with God and turns our hearts and minds toward His character, grace, love, and mercy instead of the disease and the challenges it brings.

Being open about our struggles and fears allows God to work through our lives unobstructed. In these moments of vulnerability, we experience His grace most powerfully. When we let down our guards, we allow God to heal our wounds, renew our spirits, and guide us according to His perfect purpose and plan.

Let us be encouraged to embrace vulnerability in our spiritual lives. In prayer, we shouldn't hold back. Scripture tells us to pray confidently and boldly (Hebrews 4:16). Knowing He listens and cares for us, we can fully share our hearts with God. In worship, we can let our praises rise from a place of sincerity, even when words are hard to find, or our singing is decidedly off-key.

A CLOSING THOUGHT

Vulnerability is not a sign of weakness, but a pathway to deeper intimacy with God. As we work through the ups and downs of this disease, may our time be marked by openness with God—allowing His presence to fill, reshape, and lead us into a deeper, more intimate relationship with Him.

REFLECTION

Take some time to read Psalm 34:18 and revisit Hebrews 4:15-16.

- Describe a time when you felt "crushed."

- Were you able to be open and turn to God for help during this time?

- Make a list in your journal of how the Lord has helped you in this situation.

- How does the fact that Jesus knows every emotion and hurt help you to come boldly to Him in prayer and worship?

PART FOUR

Embracing Moments of Joy

*Now may the God of hope fill you with all joy
and peace in believing, that you may abound
in hope by the power of the Holy Spirit.*

ROMANS 15:13

DAY 16

Harmonizing Hope

It was December. The side effects of a recent chemotherapy treatment hit with full force. It was undoubtedly stressful, but through this difficulty, I discovered a source of comfort: Christmas music. As I struggled, the melodies of Christmas became soothing reminders of the incarnation. Jesus left the wonders of heaven to be with us in our darkest moments. He is the One surpassing all darkness, here to rescue and save us.

The timeless carol "Joy to the World" took on a profound meaning. The words resonated with the deep emotions we should feel about the incarnation. The song also served as a life lesson, urging me to embrace a joyful heart despite the circumstances. I realized afresh what Jesus has done in His infinite love and what remarkable things He will continue to do as His joy, hope, and peace replace our sadness, fear, and discouragement.

When circumstances seem overwhelmingly negative,

we can easily assume bad attitudes. However, I've realized we don't have to succumb to negativity. Jesus gave us something on the inside that surpasses anything on the outside (1 John 4:4). This understanding should empower us to live with joyful hearts, to appreciate the power of His love even through adversity.

In the face of challenging circumstances like cancer, chemotherapy, and side effects, finding joy can be a profound testimony of our lives with Jesus. The ability to choose joy despite our difficulties is a powerful witness. The reassurance found in Philippians 4:4 becomes a guiding light in the darkest moments: "Always be *full of joy* in the Lord. I say it again—rejoice!" (NLT, emphasis mine). Paul found joy, not in his circumstances or in what he had, but in who he knew: Jesus. Pastor Roger Ellsworth wrote on this theme:

> This joy-intoxicated man [the apostle Paul] could not stress too much the importance of his fellow believers rejoicing, but, as always, the cause of the Christians' rejoicing is the Lord. Paul is not calling here for some kind of general, happy optimism that has no basis. There are no reasons for rejoicing without the Lord, but with him there is no end to such reasons.[1]

Joy is a choice. It is a decision to secure ourselves in what only God can give us. Circumstances are fleeting and subject to change. However, the joy that emanates from a deep-rooted connection with the Lord and understanding that He guides our steps can become a constant…if we choose to receive it.

A CLOSING THOUGHT

Joy is not a fleeting emotion but a resilient, sustaining, uplifting force. It comes from the assurance that, through Jesus the Messiah, we find the strength to endure, overcome, and, ultimately, experience an exultation that lifts us beyond our circumstances.

REFLECTION

Read James 1:2 and Galatians 5:22.

- Journal your thoughts about this definition of joy: "Joy comes only from God. Joy is a supernatural delight in the Person, purposes, and people of God."[2]
- How would you differentiate happiness from genuine joy?
- What about joy makes this our aim, rather than happiness?

DAY 17

Embracing Joyful Gratitude

There have been moments during my cancer journey that have caused me to be alone. I've turned off my phone and taken advantage of the time. Surprisingly, the solitude has been more than okay. As I've coped with this disease, solitude has become an opportunity to reflect and celebrate the profound gratitude I have for my family, for my doctors, and most importantly, for Jesus and how He's changed my life.

Gratitude, like joy, has the power to renew our perspectives, offering a glimmer of hope amid adversity. During life's most challenging chapters, when the weight of uncertainty and the trials of cancer press heavily upon us, we also receive a profound invitation: an invitation to cultivate and seek out gratitude and a joyful heart.

Psalm 105 is one of my favorite psalms. Written by

David, king and songwriter, the first 15 verses of this beautiful psalm are also contained in 1 Chronicles 16:8-22, when David returned the ark of the covenant to Jerusalem. The first five verses of Psalm 105 in *The Message* translation read:

> Hallelujah!
> Thank GOD! Pray to him by name!
> Tell everyone you meet what he has done!
> Sing him songs, belt out hymns,
> translate his wonders into music!
> Honor his holy name with Hallelujahs,
> you who seek GOD. Live a happy life!
> Keep your eyes open for GOD,
>   watch for his works;
> be alert for signs of his presence.
> Remember the world of wonders he
>   has made,
> his miracles, and the verdicts he's
>   rendered.

You might be wondering: *How can I thank God as I deal with this awful disease and treatment?* Expressing gratitude to God can be a profound and personal journey. Genesis 29–30 gives us an example of gratitude despite adverse circumstances. In this story, Jacob unknowingly married

Leah, Rachel's older sister, as a result of his father-in-law's deception. Jacob loved Rachel and had asked for her hand in marriage, but he found himself married instead to a woman he did not love. Leah, hoping to earn his affection, bore Jacob many sons despite being unloved. However, she ultimately found her worth in being grateful to God.

No doubt, Leah lived a problematic life and had every reason to be bitter and discouraged. However, the ancient Jewish writings in the Talmud portray her as a shining example of gratitude.[1]

Leah's fourth son was beyond what she had anticipated receiving.[2] Genesis 29:35 says, "Once again Leah became pregnant and gave birth to another son. She named him Judah, for she said, 'Now I will praise the Lord!' And then she stopped having children" (NLT).

Leah's gratitude for this child was profound and sincere, as he was an unanticipated gift from God. Acknowledging him as an extra blessing, she named him *Judah*, which means "praise" in Hebrew.

Recognizing that she was unloved by Jacob, as well as the resulting heartbreak, could have kept her in a very negative place. However, Leah turned things around. She experienced God's grace and mercy, and in the words of Rabbi Shai Held, she "express[ed] gratitude even and especially amid profound sorrow and enduring disappointment."[3]

A CLOSING THOUGHT

Gratitude shifts our focus from what we lack (emotionally, physically, or spiritually) to the abundance we possess in the Lord. A thankful perspective cultivates joy as we become more aware of and appreciative of our blessings.

REFLECTION

Slowly read Psalms 92 and 105.

- How does the psalmist emphasize the value of giving thanks?
- In your journal, list ways you can show your thanks to God.
- In what ways can you show gratitude to other people? Commit to showing gratitude regularly and bringing joy to yourself and others.

DAY 18

Finding Shalom in the Stillness

My journey through cancer has unfolded a chapter of profound personal reformation and significant spiritual learning. As is true for many, I've encountered myriad side effects as I've moved from medications and injections to chemotherapy. Among these, fatigue has been a constant companion, weaving itself into my daily life. Sometimes fatigue is a shadow in the background, and at other times, a demanding presence at the forefront.

Before my cancer began, I thrived on action and engagement. My enthusiasm for understanding and applying personality and temperament tests fueled me and my work culture. My top strength, being an "activator," encapsulates me perfectly: a drive for action, making things happen, and turning plans into reality.

Relentless fatigue has offended my very nature. Yet,

in this challenging season, God has been my teacher, revealing insights into the depths of His Word and the power of living within His leadership and guidance. In the meantime, two Hebrew words have become beacons of hope and strength: *shalom* and *damam*.

Shalom extends far beyond mere peace or absence of conflict. *Shalom* encompasses completeness, soundness, and welfare—the elements of life unmarred by deficiency.[1] It signifies a godly grace expressed as tranquility and security in one's life. Isaiah 26:3 beautifully captures this idea: "You will keep him in perfect peace [*shalom*], whose mind is stayed on You, because he trusts in You." While battling cancer, *shalom* has become a cherished state of being, an anchor amid the storm, reminding me of the wholeness found in God's presence, promises, plan, and purpose.

Damam, meanwhile, invites me into a realm of quietude and rest, a stillness that transcends mere physical repose.[2] Psalm 37:7 encourages, "Rest [*damam*] in the Lord, and wait patiently for Him." This call to stillness—to welcome silence, to cease striving—has been a profound challenge for someone driven to action. Yet, in this stillness, I've found a new form of action: a focused, deliberate turning of my heart and mind toward the Lord, as I wait on Him with expectancy and trust.

The lessons from God and His Word touch my core, shifting my understanding of action and purpose. I've learned the value of embracing tranquility and rest, seeing the Lord in the stillness, and finding deep joy in simply spending time in His presence. An "activator" finds profound fulfillment in *damam*—in the rest, the waiting, the listening.

The benefit of this rest and waiting on Him is *shalom*. Psalm 29:11 reminds us that "God makes his people strong. God gives his people peace [*shalom*]" (msg). I've learned that strength comes not necessarily from my actions, but from my resting in Him. And, when I rest in Him, I find *shalom*: inner peace, joy, and contentment.

A CLOSING THOUGHT

Despite our circumstances, we can stand firm on the solid ground of *shalom*. Quiet strength from resting (*damam*) in God empowers us. When we keep our minds focused on God and trust Him, He will keep us in perfect peace and rest, resulting in unimaginable joy.

REFLECTION

Read John 14:27.

- How does godly peace differ from the worldly understanding of peace?
- In what ways can believers practically experience and show this peace in their daily lives, especially in times of trouble and uncertainty?

Read Exodus 33:14.

- How does this assurance from God to Moses reflect His relationship with His people?
- What implications does this have for understanding the concept of rest and the Lord's support of cancer patients and caregivers?
- In your journal, reflect on how God's presence brings about a sense of rest or peace, even in trials or life's wilderness seasons.

DAY 19

Two of Us

Paul McCartney and John Lennon wrote a song entitled "Two of Us." The song, mostly from McCartney's perspective, chronicles the fun days he and his wife Linda had "riding nowhere" as they joyfully journeyed in their car through the English countryside without a specific destination.

The song reminds me of the relationship between the patient and their caregiver. Together, they navigate the vast and often uncertain landscape of health challenges like two companions traveling through life's zigzagging paths. The two work together to manage incredibly challenging circumstances—traveling the road, enjoying the countryside as Paul and Linda did, or sometimes getting lost. Speaking about his wife, McCartney said, "She loved getting lost. And she pointed out to me quite rightly that there would always be a sign somewhere saying 'London,' so we'd just follow that."[1]

Not knowing where the road leads is sometimes part of the journey and can lead to joy. McCartney's reflection on his adventures with Linda offers hope: There's always a way back, a sign leading you home, reminding you that getting a little lost isn't necessarily a bad thing, especially when you're sharing the journey with someone who has your welfare as a patient as their highest priority.

With Jesus, we are never genuinely lost. First John 3:1 reminds us, "See how very much our Father loves us, for he calls us his children, and that is what we are!" (NLT). John points out that we are not merely called the children of God; we *are* the children of God. Nothing compares to God's love for us; because of His faithful love, we are never lost.

Balancing life challenges, managing disease, and enjoying life are crucial for patients and caregivers. Integrating activities that bring joy and relaxation into one's daily routine is essential, helping reduce stress and improve overall well-being.

My caregiver is my wife, and we have found that we can have enjoyable times together. We also try to laugh and find humor whenever possible. Although we can both be serious, finding things to laugh at uplifts our moods and helps us set aside the rigors of this disease. Sometimes we laugh at life's moments; other times, a funny movie provides much-needed humor. Other times we feel lost, but God points us back home to His Word, will, and ways.

When we feel lost, we turn to prayer and God's Word to show us the way back home. When we stop and pray, we find a calmness and peace that overcomes the challenges of our circumstances.

A joyful spirit is the anthem that keeps us moving forward, focusing on the possibilities rather than the obstacles. This journey is ever-changing; we must be open to adapting and adjusting our course along the way. This is not a sign of defeat, but of strength and resilience.

A CLOSING THOUGHT

You and your caregiver can navigate the challenges of chronic illness with joy, togetherness, and the ever-present grace of God. Set about creating a life of resilience, love, and unyielding hope—reminders that, even in the face of life's uncertainties, you can together find your way back home to a place of peace and joy.

REFLECTION

Make the time to thank those who provide your care: your doctors, nurses, and caregivers. Your show of gratitude toward them will not only brighten their days but will also give you joy.

Read Psalms 107:4 and 119:176.

- In your journal, describe a time when you felt lost.

- What brought you back home?

- Have you ever felt lost or far from God?

- How does knowing you are His child, under His sovereign care, help you to return home to Him?

DAY 20

Finding Joy Despite All That's Bad

In a sermon titled "What Is the Secret to Joy in Life?" Pastor Rick Warren taught:

> Most people don't know the two secrets of joy, but I'm going to give them to you… Number one is get the focus off myself. The more you focus on you, the more miserable you're going to be…[Second], shift your inward focus to outward focus—it's all about God and serving others.[1]

Cancer is an awful disease. According to the World Health Organization, it "is a leading cause of death worldwide, accounting for nearly 10 million deaths in 2020, or nearly one in six deaths."[2] That's bad. Yet having an attitude of joy rather than discouragement, fear, and doubt will refill your emotional gas tank.

Job 1:20-22 shows us how we can have joy despite dire circumstances:

> Then Job arose, tore his robe, and shaved his head; and he fell to the ground and worshiped. And he said: "Naked I came from my mother's womb, and naked shall I return there. The LORD gave, and the LORD has taken away; blessed be the name of the LORD." In all this Job did not sin nor charge God with wrong.

After losing his property, his health, and his children, Job worshiped God. When nothing around him made sense, Job worshiped God. He took the focus away from his loss and himself and decided to focus outwardly on the Lord. In so doing, Job released his grief to God. Job never lost faith in God's sovereignty (Romans 8:28; Job 23:10)—the God who could give and take away. He knew his God. He stood firm amid horrific circumstances and reflected on God's goodness.

Second Corinthians 11:23-29 gives us an idea of the dreadful circumstances in which the apostle Paul found himself. In these few verses, Paul detailed his numerous sufferings for Jesus, including imprisonments, countless beatings, and near-death experiences. He endured being lashed, beaten with rods, stoned, and shipwrecked. He faced dangers from rivers, robbers, his people (the Jews), and Gentiles. Additionally, he experienced hardships such as hunger, thirst, cold, and exposure and felt daily pressure because of his concern for all the churches. Despite these trials, his commitment to spreading the gospel never wavered.

Paul's focus was not on himself or his circumstances. He focused on God and the gospel message God had given him to spread. In Ephesians 3, Paul emphasized a remarkable truth: He wasn't caught off guard by his suffering; rather, he was amazed by the joy he found while in it. Suffering for Jesus is challenging, but every hardship is profoundly worth it for the joy and purpose it brings. Paul was a prisoner awaiting a Roman trial. Under house arrest, he was free to roam the house during the day but chained to a Roman guard at night. Yet, despite all the bad things that happened to him, Paul, like Job, found joy in the Lord. He even wrote the letter to the Philippians, which was all about joy!

A CLOSING THOUGHT

When we endure hardships with joy, faith, and confidence rather than bitterness, complaints, and anger, we become powerful witnesses to God's love and honor Jesus in a profound way. Our steadfastness in adversity shines as a testament to His grace and strength in our lives.

REFLECTION

Read Psalms 69:32 and 145:1.

- In your journal, note how you can worship God despite your circumstances.
- How do you think worshiping God will help you find joy and contentment?

Read 1 Thessalonians 5:18.

- How could the apostle Paul give thanks in all circumstances? (Here's a clue: The verse says *in* all circumstances, not *for* all circumstances.)
- How can focusing on God and others refill your emotional gas tank?

PART FIVE

Finding Purpose in the Journey

*I know the thoughts that I think toward you,
says the L*ORD*, thoughts of peace and
not of evil, to give you a future and a hope.*

JEREMIAH 29:11

DAY 21

Finding Purpose Through Difficulty

Perhaps you have heard the oft-repeated idea that the two most important days in your life are the day you were born and the day you discover why.[1]

Similarly, we may ask, "Why am I here?" Each of us wants to know our purpose, yet enduring the ups and downs of cancer and treatment may obscure our view of God's intent for our lives.

So how can our sense of purpose be reenergized when we're facing difficulty? The life of the Old Testament patriarch Joseph may give us some clues.

Joseph, one of the twelve sons of Jacob, was favored by his father, which stirred up jealousy among his brothers. This favoritism, symbolized by the gift of a multicolored coat, led his brothers to conspire against him (Genesis 37:3-4). They initially planned to kill Joseph, but they sold him into slavery, which landed him in Egypt (Genesis 37:18-20, 27-28). Despite his unfortunate circumstances, Joseph's integrity and God's favor led him to a position of responsibility in the household of Potiphar, an Egyptian official (Genesis 39:2-5). However, after rejecting the advances of Potiphar's wife (Genesis 39:11-15), Joseph was falsely accused and imprisoned (Genesis 39:19-20).

In prison, Joseph's ability to interpret dreams brought him to the attention of Pharaoh, who was troubled by disturbing dreams (Genesis 41:14-16). Joseph interpreted Pharaoh's dreams, predicting seven years of abundance followed by seven years of famine (Genesis 41:29-32). Impressed by his wisdom, Pharaoh appointed Joseph as Egypt's second-in-command, overseeing surplus grain storage and distribution (Genesis 41:39-45). During the famine, Joseph's brothers came to Egypt to buy food but did not recognize him (Genesis 42:1-8). After a series of interactions, Joseph revealed his identity and forgave them, attributing his hardships to God's plan to save many lives (Genesis 45:4-15). Ultimately, Joseph's journey from betrayal to prominence exemplifies themes of purpose, resilience, trusting God's plan, and forgiveness.

Highlighting Joseph's story, Messianic Rabbi Jason Sobel wrote, "When Joseph was in the pit and the prison, it appeared the Lord had forgotten him. In His perfect timing, however, God brought Joseph out and into his place of divine calling."[2]

God worked powerfully in Joseph's life; He is working in our lives too. God has a plan and a purpose for each of us, even as we navigate the difficult conditions of this disease. Joseph's trust and relationship with God increased amid each circumstance he faced. He could see God's hand at work—just as we can if we are willing to look for it.

What we experience can be painful. Yet God is with us through the pain. He is weaving a plan for us that will be for our good and the good of others if we keep Him in focus. How? By being in His Word and by praying and asking Him to help us not merely see the short term, but also the long term. Joseph remained focused on the Lord and rose from the pit to the palace.

A CLOSING THOUGHT

Just as God had a plan for Joseph, guiding him from betrayal and hardship to a position of power where he could save many lives, He also has a unique and purposeful plan for each of us. Despite our challenges, we can trust that God works behind the scenes to bring about His good and perfect will.

REFLECTION

Read Proverbs 16:9 and 19:21. Read Psalm 37:23.

- In what ways do you think having plans is good for you?

- How should the Lord's counsel affect the plans you've made?

- When and why might you find yourself struggling to believe that the Lord's plans are truly better than yours? What ultimately gives you confidence in the Lord?

DAY 22

Trusting God's Plan

Several years ago, I joined a company with significant financial issues. The company wasn't profitable and had severe cash flow problems. One morning, I entered the building early and found the CEO's light on. Upon entering his office, I discovered he was reading his Bible. He pointed to the verse over which he was praying, Jeremiah 29:11 (the key verse for this section of the devotional). That morning, we committed to praying this verse daily, and as we did, things began to change for the company. Thanks to the Lord's guidance, the company turned around. God did have a plan for us: not to take us out of business, but to make us whole and substantial so we could continue ministering.

Chapter 29 of the Old Testament book of Jeremiah contains a collection of letters written to the Jewish exiles living in Babylon. The prophet wrote the letters to comfort the troubled, homesick Jews who had been taken from their homes by the Babylonians and then forcibly moved into a pagan culture over 800 miles away. They were exiled to a land of people who did not worship the Jewish God, *Yahweh*.

The prophet encouraged the exiles to settle into their new environment, start families, plant gardens, and put down roots (verses 5-7). He warned them about the pagan gods and the false teachings they'd encounter as they lived in the Babylonian culture. Then Jeremiah wrote,

> "For I know the plans I have for you," says the LORD. "They are plans for good and not for disaster, to give you a future and a hope" (Jeremiah 29:11 NLT).

The people must have thought, *What plans? What hope? What kind of future do we have in this place?* They lived in the pain of exile and distress, torn away from families, friends, and their homeland.

In this letter, we find God giving His people a promise: He has a purpose and plan to bring a future and hope. Pastor Warren Wiersbe wrote,

> God makes His plans for His people, and they are good plans that ultimately bring

hope and peace. Therefore, there is no need to be afraid or discouraged.[1]

Today, as we live with cancer, God is saying the same thing to us. Despite our discouragement, pain, fear, and maybe even feelings that we have been exiled, God has a purpose and a plan for us. As I've battled cancer, God has clearly shown me a renewed purpose and plan. As I went to the oncologist's office, I saw people who were hurting and who needed to hear an encouraging word or merely see a smile. I also saw doctors, nurses, and technicians working intently to care for their patients. God gave me a fresh purpose: to be kind and encouraging, and to talk about His love and grace to anyone I encountered. Pam and I call it "dropping seeds," as we both committed to this renewed plan of action despite the personal challenges brought on by the disease.

Do you see God working in your life to create a new purpose and plan? Take time out to be alone with Him, and let Him give you a future and hope with His counsel for a new or refreshed direction.

A CLOSING THOUGHT

God has a plan, and that plan is good. Our question is: "How do I access it? Other people seem to receive guidance. How can I?" I know no better time to answer these questions than now, as we enter the next room in God's Great House and pray, "Thy will be done."[2]

REFLECTION

Read Psalms 25:4-5 and 139:1-8.

- In what ways has God prepared you for this journey?

- How does the promise of Jeremiah 29:11 impact your understanding of God's intentions for your life, especially during difficult times?

- Reflecting on these two passages from the Psalms, consider a time when you felt uncertain about your future. How might these verses have provided comfort or direction?

- How did you experience God's plan and guidance during that season?

DAY 23

The Refining Fire

Sometimes we need to discover God's purpose for our lives. We seek Him through prayer and His Word as He uncovers His plans, even as we face challenges.

Pam and I have faced many refining fires that fortified our faith. I was recently diagnosed with a second cancer (B-cell lymphoma), and my first chemotherapy treatment put me down. Less than a week after the initial treatment, I stood in the bathroom, and everything went black. I fell, hit my chin on the counter, and tumbled against an unforgiving wall, severely bruising my back. Pam called EMS, I blacked out again, and EMS took me to the hospital for a twelve-day stay. Because the lymphoma had depleted my immune system, the hospital doctors put me in isolation, and no visitors were allowed. Pam wasn't feeling well, so we spent several days without seeing each other. I was scared and alone.

I could have responded to this challenge in several

ways, from anger to depression to discouragement. But instead, I read Psalm 46 and other psalms, mainly penned by David, in which he and the psalmists expressed their sorrow but chose to trust God despite the circumstances. I listened to my favorite pastors online and learned much about God's love, grace, patience, and mercy. I prayed frequently. And I chose to encourage and affirm all the hospital staff with words of thankfulness and testimony to the Lord.

Looking back, I recognize that God's purpose was to take me through refining fire. God had a plan and purpose for me losing consciousness. The hospital stay enabled me to find ways to learn, to become closer to Him, and to drop seeds of encouragement and faith to a group of people caring diligently for their patients.

The apostle Peter also needed some refining. God refined the often-outspoken apostle through his denial of Jesus and subsequent restoration. This humbling experience transformed him from a rash and impulsive disciple into a bold and faithful leader in the early church (Luke 22:54-62; John 21:15-19).

Later in his life, Peter wrote:

> I know how great this makes you feel, even though you have to put up with every kind of aggravation in the meantime. Pure gold

put in the fire comes out of it proved pure; genuine faith put through this suffering comes out proved genuine. When Jesus wraps this all up, it's your faith, not your gold, that God will have on display as evidence of his victory (1 Peter 1:6-7 MSG).

Peter eventually understood that trials refine our faith like fire and uncover the beauty and strength that emerge as gold. Going through life's refining fires—trusting God's purpose without comprehending it—increases our faith. We can come to this same understanding. Instead of being angry or upset, we can embrace the trial and watch our faith in the Lord maturing and growing.

A CLOSING THOUGHT

Understanding God's purpose in our fiery trials is crucial because it gives us hope and perspective, assuring us that our suffering is not in vain. Recognizing that God is refining and strengthening our character and faith through these challenges helps us trust His sovereign plan, deepens our faith, and prepares us for more incredible things in His service.

REFLECTION

Read Job 38, where we see God responding to the horrific circumstances Job endured in previous chapters.

- How can asking "why" prevent us from seeing God's purpose?

- How does asking "why" sometimes weaken our trust in God?

- How does discovering God's purpose without asking "why" strengthen our faith?

Read 2 Corinthians 1:3-4.

- Describe a time you felt that God was putting you through a fiery trial.

- Review and journal what you think God's purpose was for the trial. What did the trial teach you?

DAY 24

The Good Shepherd

When I read Psalm 23, I find David's statement about walking through "the valley of the shadow of death" a poignant and powerful metaphor for our lives' darkest and most challenging times. For those of us battling cancer, this valley is a place fraught with physical pain, emotional turmoil, and spiritual questioning. Yet within these shadows, a profound promise from our Good Shepherd brings comfort and purpose to every step we take.

Psalm 23:4 declares,

> Even though I walk through the valley of the shadow of death, I will fear no evil, for You are with me: Your rod and Your staff comfort me (TLV).

This verse captures the Good Shepherd's heart: He

walks beside us in our darkest and most challenging moments, providing protection, purpose, and guidance.

I've found that God's presence is the cornerstone of my comfort during difficult times. Knowing God is with me transforms my perspective. He reassures me, even when the path ahead seems insurmountable. God's presence is the constant source of strength. God is always with me, reminding me that He is intimately aware of my struggles and actively involved in my journey. He guides me toward His purpose through everything I endure.

The imagery of the rod and staff in Psalm 23:4 is rich with meaning. The rod symbolizes God's protection, warding off our fears. The staff represents His guidance, gently directing us down the right path. As we deal with cancer, we can be assured that God is actively defending us against spiritual and emotional harm and guiding us toward His purposes.

One of the most challenging aspects of cancer is finding purpose amid suffering. Yet our Good Shepherd is not only our Comforter, but also the One who infuses our journey with meaning. Romans 8:28 reminds us, "We know that all things work together for good to those who love God, to those who are the called according to *His* purpose." This verse encourages us to trust that God is using our experiences, even the painful ones, to accomplish His greater plan.

Our suffering can become powerful testaments to God's faithfulness. When we walk through the valley with faith and trust, and when others can see the strength and hope that comes from our relationship with God, they may learn to trust in His purpose as well. Our journeys can inspire and encourage those around us, drawing them closer to the Good Shepherd.

God's comfort doesn't eliminate our pain, but it provides a profound assurance that we are cared for and loved. In the valley, as we lean on Him, we often experience the deepest intimacy with God.

A CLOSING THOUGHT

As we navigate the challenging circumstances of cancer, let us embrace the care of our Good Shepherd. May we trust in His presence, rely on His protection and guidance, and seek His purpose for us at every step of our journey. Remember, our Shepherd leads us through the valleys and toward green pastures and still waters, promising restoration and peace.

REFLECTION

Everything God asks us to do is for our good. He is the Good Shepherd.

Now carefully read Psalm 23 and Isaiah 43:1-2.

- What do these verses tell you about God?

- How can this assurance of God's presence, purpose, and protection help you face the waters and rivers of life with courage and faith?

DAY 25

Letting Your Light Shine

During a battle with cancer, one can easily become overwhelmed by the accompanying physical, relational, emotional, and spiritual challenges. Yet even in our darkest moments, Jesus calls us to shine our lights before others, demonstrating God's love, purpose, and grace. In Matthew 5:13-16, Jesus said:

> Let me tell you why you are here. You're here to be salt-seasoning that brings out the God-flavors of this earth. If you lose your saltiness, how will people taste godliness? You've lost your usefulness and will end up in the garbage. Here's another way to put it: You're here to be light, bringing out the God-colors in the world. God is not a secret to be kept. We're going public with this, as public as a city on a hill. If I make you

light-bearers, you don't think I'm going to hide you under a bucket, do you? I'm putting you on a light stand. Now that I've put you there on a hilltop, on a light stand—shine! Keep open house; be generous with your lives. By opening up to others, you'll prompt people to open up with God, this generous Father in heaven (MSG).

Jesus identifies His people as the world's light, a powerful declaration that surpasses our circumstances. Even as we face cancer trials, we possess a light that can shine brightly. This light is not dependent on our physical strength or emotional stability; it is rooted in our faith in Jesus and His work within us. Our light is a testament to God's love, grace, and purpose—shining through our fight with cancer.

One of the most powerful ways to let our light shine is by focusing on others. Cancer can make life feel insular, as pain and fear often draw our attention inward. However, we can find renewed resolve and strength when we shift our focus to those around us. Acts of kindness, words of encouragement, and simply being present for others are potent ways to demonstrate God's love.

We also need to consider the people in our lives who might be struggling. Despite our challenges, our willingness to reach out and support those people can be significant. Whether you help a fellow patient, a caregiver, or a family member, your light can brighten their path, reminding them that God's love endures despite the circumstances they face.

In addition to demonstrating God's love, letting our lights shine involves living with purpose. Cancer may disrupt our plans, but it cannot extinguish God's intention for us. Hebrews 11:39-40 underscores this thought: "These were all commended for their faith, yet none of them received what had been promised, *since God had planned something better*" (NIV, emphasis mine). Pastor Jon Courson wrote,

> The Lord lives in our hearts. He walks with us every moment of every day. He gives direction to us whenever we take time to stop and listen.[1]

A CLOSING THOUGHT

You can take heart and be encouraged. Your light is a gift from God, meant to shine brightly even during trials. By letting your light shine, you reflect God's love, purpose, and grace and find renewed strength and joy in focusing on the needs of others. God is using your journey to bring light to a world in need.

REFLECTION

Read John 12:36 and Luke 14:34-35.

- What is your understanding of the concept of becoming "children of light"?

- What characteristics or behaviors might define someone who lives as a child of light?

- The ancient world used salt for preservation and flavor. How can we, as Christians, be agents of preservation and bring flavor to the world around us, especially when we are enduring challenging circumstances?

PART SIX

Celebrating Small Victories

Thanks be to God! He gives us the victory through our Lord Jesus Christ.

1 CORINTHIANS 15:57 NIV

DAY 26

Keep Going

We often overlook the small victories, fixating instead on the grand accomplishments. We want to lose 20 pounds and don't celebrate the pound we lost yesterday. We miss a putt for par and forget the incredible chip shot that got us on the green. Yet we should remind ourselves that significant achievements require time and persistent effort. Remember the saying, "Rome wasn't built in a day"? Our ability to keep going despite the frustration and pain of cancer comes from taking consistent small steps in the right direction.

In the Bible, we see this principle reflected in the life of King David. Before he became the renowned King of Israel, David faithfully tended his father's sheep, defeated Goliath, and endured years of trials and tribulations. Each small victory prepared him for the greater purpose God had for him. David's story reminds us that our daily efforts and seemingly minor achievements are essential building blocks for God's plan.

Small victories are the milestones that mark our progress toward a larger goal. The wins may seem insignificant, but they are vital to our growth and motivation. No matter how small, every step we take brings us closer to our destination. Celebrating our progress builds our confidence, strengthens our resolve, and gives us the courage to face wearisome challenges.

Besides David, the Bible has several examples of individuals who experienced small victories that led to significant achievements. Moses, for instance, led the children of Israel out of Egypt step-by-step, facing numerous challenges along the way. With God's help, each hurdle he overcame brought him closer to fulfilling God's promise of delivering His people to the promised land.

Proverbs 16:9 tells us, "We can make our plans, but the LORD determines our steps" (NLT). This verse encourages us to trust that each small, God-directed movement is part of an overarching journey. We acknowledge God's hand in our progress by celebrating our small victories and moving forward with Him.

When I returned home from a hospital visit, my legs were weakened. I knew I needed to strengthen them, but I could not walk much. I set a goal for distance using a step tracker and celebrated each time I accomplished more movement than the previous day, even if it was only by ten steps. Celebrating each small victory gave me hope and confidence that I could achieve my larger goal. I could have been disappointed at my weakness and my lack of immediate results, but I knew God was at work in every step I took. I could celebrate His faithfulness and guidance toward my goal.

We can also enjoy and appreciate the journey rather than focusing on the destination. Amid our journey with the Lord, we will grow, learn, and experience His grace. When we embrace each step of the process, we allow ourselves to experience God's blessing.

Paul wrote in Philippians 1:6, "Being confident of this, that he who began a good work in you will carry it on to completion until the day of Christ Jesus" (NIV). This assurance reminds us that God is continually at work in us, shaping us through every small challenge and conquest. We can find joy in each small victory by trusting His process.

As we fight cancer, we should take time to reflect on the progress we've made, no matter how seemingly insignificant. We can cultivate an attitude of gratitude, thanking God for every small victory and the lessons learned along the way. We can also encourage and inspire fellow patients, nurses, and doctors by sharing our small triumphs with them.

A CLOSING THOUGHT

Every small victory, kindness, step of faith, and determined act brings us closer to God's vision. To embrace and celebrate small victories is essential, knowing these wins are significant milestones on our paths to confidence, hope, and a better understanding of God's plan for our lives.

REFLECTION

Take a few moments to read Proverbs 20:24 and 2 Thessalonians 1:11.

- In your journal, list some small victories you've experienced. Prayerfully thank God for those small victories and how He's leading you to the goal of perfecting your faith.

DAY 27

Resetting Expectations

As I write this, I'm going through my second experience with chemotherapy. I've learned that the three weeks between sessions can be challenging and insightful. Typically, I have one bad week, one fair week, and one good week. During the three weeks between treatments, I've rested, worked, and been thankful for how the treatments kill cancer cells. I've also done quite a bit of thinking. One thought I've dwelled upon is how my patience has improved, but my nagging thoughts have been about expectations.

I have a lot of expectations for myself. As a sports and athletics person, I always expected to pitch a no-hitter or hit the game-winning home run. I fully expected to throw touchdown passes or hit the perfect jump shot. When I was playing football as a freshman in high school, those expectations ended after I suffered a traumatic knee injury. Not being one to accept defeat, I tried basketball and baseball, only to have two additional knee injuries that ended my athletic career.

I have not been the sole author of these expectations. We all know and have experienced the myriad expectations others place upon us: the expectations of parents, employers, ministries. Many of these expectations are well-meant, but each one threatens to replace our primary call to do the Father's will.

I've learned that we need to recalibrate during extreme challenges, wholly setting aside our expectations and exchanging them for God's expectations. Through this process, we will experience the small victories that come from turning everything over to Him. He will do what He's promised to do.

Psalm 27:14 tells us, "Wait on the Lord; be of good courage, and He shall strengthen your heart; wait I say, on the Lord!" We should work with God toward His goals for us. He is the best cheerleader and encourager we could have as we reset our expectations and celebrate small victories. As the psalmist wrote, we should wait, hope, expect, endure, and be brave (and I'd add celebrate) during challenging times.

I've needed to rethink my expectations. Some days I rest, or Pam and I do something fun. Other times I work on writing projects. I try not to set too many expectations because, in an instant, things can change. Instead,

I trust God for the day and celebrate the small things He's doing in my life.

Satan uses difficult situations to steal our joy. If, during challenges like cancer or cancer treatment, we only expect the worst, we subvert the positive focus we need to heal. We can't change our circumstances, but we can change our outlook. We can enjoy fewer or no expectations. We can enjoy small victories.

Pastor Jentezen Franklin said, "Don't let the big issues hold you hostage. Instead, walk in victory over the little things. The little wins will add up. Every incredible journey is one mile at a time."[1]

A CLOSING THOUGHT

We can reset our expectations, trust God's plan instead of our own, and celebrate our small victories. We can't let the enemy rob us of our joy, not for one hour or one day. Reset and celebrate.

REFLECTION

Many people adopt an attitude that says, "Until everything is perfect, I can't truly celebrate or be happy."

Now read 1 Samuel 14:24-29. King Saul's foolish oath

prevented the soldiers from receiving the small victory God put right before them.

- Reflect on 1 Samuel 14. How can you shift your mindset to celebrate small victories and be grateful, even when your expectations are not fully met?

- In your journal, write some practical steps you can take to celebrate small victories, even when they fall short of your expectations.

- What expectations do you think God has for you?

DAY 28

From Grumbling to Gratitude

As we navigate cancer and various treatments, it's easy to feel overwhelmed and succumb to weariness, complaints, and grumbling.

I recently found myself in this very predicament during what was supposed to be my "good week" post-chemotherapy. The side effects took their toll, and I wallowed in frustration and discontent. I turned to prayer and comfort in Scripture in this moment of distress. I found guidance from the apostle Paul's words in Philippians 2:14-16.

Paul's exhortation to "do all things without complaining and disputing" walloped me (Philippians 2:14). His words reminded me that while feeling the urge to grumble may be natural, grumbling ultimately serves no purpose beyond keeping me stuck in negativity. Reflecting on the children of Israel's 40 years of wandering due to their complaints in the wilderness, I realized the destructive power of discontentment.

Thanks to the apostle's words, I recognized that my complaints were falling on deaf ears. Even more, my attitude was a personal offense to God. By grumbling, I disregarded His sovereignty, provision, and ability to grant me the grace, peace, and strength needed to endure the various challenges before me.

In that moment of realization, I consciously shifted my perspective. Instead of dwelling on the negatives, I chose to "rejoice always and delight in [my] faith," as urged by 1 Thessalonians 5:16 (AMP). I tried to look for the silver linings in every situation, refusing to let a critical spirit hinder the work of the Holy Spirit in my life.

I cannot overstate the power of small victories in our lives. These little breakthroughs help us see our journeys from different perspectives. Every little step forward, no matter how minor it may seem, is a testament to God's work and gives us a reason to celebrate. Focusing on the positive shifts our perspectives from grumbling to gratitude.

Jesus tells us in Matthew 5:14-16 that we are the light of the world. We let our light shine before others by embracing gratitude and celebrating God's provision. Our ability to radiate God's love and goodness is directly connected to our willingness to embrace joy and thankfulness, especially as we face challenges without complaining.

We can begin a daily practice of gratitude, reflecting on the blessings and goodness of God, even during the hard times (1 Thessalonians 5:18). We can also read God's Word, trusting His promises and purpose (Hebrews 10:23). We can pray and set aside a daily devotional time. We can carve out moments throughout the day for prayer, reflection, and reading Scripture, all of which enable God's presence to infuse strength and peace into our souls. We can make a conscious decision each day to choose joy over despair, trusting in God's sovereignty and goodness regardless of circumstances.

A CLOSING THOUGHT

Let us exchange our complaints for thankfulness, grumbling for joy, and despair for hope. By embracing gratitude and celebrating small victories, we can overcome negativity and find strength, peace, and gladness in the Lord's goodness and mercy.

REFLECTION

Take time to read and study Psalm 77.

- How does this passage model gratitude as a response to trouble rather than grumbling?

- How can shifting your focus from grumbling to gratitude change your perspective on your challenges?

- How do small victories help you to see your journey through a different lens?

DAY 29

Embracing Failures and Small Victories

Cancer treatment can feel like a roller coaster of emotions, filled with triumphant highs and devastating lows. When we face the lows, it's easy to become discouraged by setbacks and failures. The Bible reminds us that even in our struggles, God is at work, shaping a story of perseverance, growth, and eternal victory. Embracing our setbacks as part of this journey shifts our focus, helping us to see the value in both our steps forward and our setbacks.

The apostle Paul provided us profound insights regarding setbacks. In Philippians 3:13-14, he wrote,

> No, dear brothers and sisters, I have not achieved it, but I focus on this one thing: Forgetting the past and looking forward to

> what lies ahead, I press on to reach the end of the race and receive the heavenly prize for which God, through Christ Jesus, is calling us (NLT).

Paul's words encourage us to not dwell on past failures or setbacks, but to keep pressing forward, focusing on the eternal goal God has set before us.

Failure and setbacks are not the end of the road but integral parts of our journey. They teach us resilience, patience, and dependence on God. When you face a setback in your cancer treatment, consider it an opportunity to lean into God's strength and trust His plan for your life. In a moment of vulnerability, you often experience the most profound growth.

The concept of small victories is crucial in this journey. Zechariah 4:10 says, "Do not despise these small beginnings, for the LORD rejoices to see the work begin" (NLT). No matter how insignificant it may seem, every small victory moves us toward a more remarkable victory in God. These small wins are reminders of God's faithfulness and presence in our lives.

As cancer patients, we must recognize and celebrate these small victories. Whether it's a good day during and after the treatments, a positive test result, or simply enough strength to get out of bed, the victories are worth celebrating. They remind us we are making progress and that God is with us every step of the way. Romans 8:1 tells us:

> Therefore, [there is] now no condemnation (no adjudging guilty of wrong) for those who are in Christ Jesus, *who live [and] walk not after the dictates of the flesh, but after the dictates of the Spirit* (AMPC).

We do not need to feel guilty, wrong, or any other negative emotion when we experience setbacks. Because we prefer ease and comfort, wanting to avoid failures or missteps seems natural—but without them, we might miss out on the lessons and growth they provide. Instead, we can shift our focus toward highlighting progress. Each day, we can reflect on the positive steps we've taken, no matter how small. To keep moving forward, we should celebrate the perseverance and courage God has granted us.

James 1:2-4 encourages us with these words:

> Dear brothers and sisters, when troubles of any kind come your way, consider it an opportunity for great joy. For you know that when your faith is tested, your endurance has a chance to grow. So let it grow, for

when your endurance is fully developed, you will be perfect and complete, needing nothing (NLT).

This New Testament passage reminds us that our trials and setbacks shape us into mature and complete Jesus followers.

A CLOSING THOUGHT

Dealing with cancer involves embracing failures and setbacks as part of God's refining process. We can celebrate small victories and recognize their significance by focusing on progress rather than perfection. We can find small victories, joy, and encouragement throughout the journey.

REFLECTION

Read 2 Corinthians 4:17-18. This passage talks about our "light and momentary troubles" that achieve for us an "eternal glory" (NIV).

- How does viewing your present difficulties in the context of eternity change your perspective on small victories and challenges?

- Share a personal experience in which this perspective helped you endure a challenging situation.

Read Revelation 3:21. In this verse, Jesus promises that those who overcome will sit with Him on His throne.

- What does it mean to overcome in the context of setbacks and small victories?
- How does Jesus's promise encourage you to persevere through difficult times?

DAY 30

Persistence and Small Wins

This section has focused on the power of small wins as we live with cancer, and one critical element of celebrating our wins is persistence. Corporate executive Saurabh Verma wrote in an article:

> Persistence plays a crucial role in achieving small wins. It can be challenging to keep going, especially when progress seems slow, or obstacles stand in your way. But those who persist keep pushing forward despite the challenges and ultimately reap the rewards of small wins.[1]

Facing cancer is daunting and demands an incredible amount of persistence. Obstacles— from the physical toll of treatments to the emotional and spiritual challenges that arise from our sickness—impede our progress. Yet a powerful truth can be found amid this problematic journey: that persistence plays a crucial role in achieving small wins. Small victories are stepping stones that can be profoundly encouraging.

The Bible speaks volumes about the importance of persistence. In Galatians 6:9, Paul wrote,

> Let us not lose heart and grow weary and faint in acting nobly and doing right, for in due time and at the appointed season we shall reap, if we do not loosen and relax our courage and faint (AMPC).

This Scripture reminds us that persistence, even when progress seems slow or imperceptible, will ultimately yield a harvest in the appointed season. For cancer patients, this means each day of perseverance, each moment of enduring treatment challenges, contributes to a more abundant, hopeful outcome.

Consider the story of Nehemiah, who was tasked with rebuilding the walls of Jerusalem. Despite facing intense opposition and numerous setbacks, he persisted. Nehemiah 4:6 states, "So we rebuilt the wall till all of it reached half its height, for the people worked with all their heart" (NIV). Each completed section of the wall was a small win, a testament to the power of persistence.

Similarly, in our battle with cancer, every small victory—every day of feeling well, or simply having the strength to smile and encourage the medical staff—is significant.

To persist in the face of cancer is not something you have to do on your own. Philippians 4:13 reminds us, "I can do all things through Christ who strengthens me." What a promise! God is our source of strength, empowering us to keep moving forward. When we feel weak, we pray to Him and let His presence renew our spirit. The journey may be arduous, but we can persevere with His strength and reap the harvest.

Jesus exemplified ultimate persistence. Despite His suffering, He remained steadfast, fulfilling His mission for our salvation. Hebrews 12:2 says, "For the joy set before him he endured the cross, scorning its shame, and sat down at the right hand of the throne of God" (NIV). Jesus's persistence through unimaginable pain brought us the most significant victory: eternal life. His example teaches us that persistence in the face of great suffering leads to profound triumph.

A CLOSING THOUGHT

Persistence is vital to achievement. Our victories, no matter how small, are significant and worthy of celebration. With God's strength, we can face each day with hope and courage. We can trust His plan, keep pushing forward, and embrace every small victory. Persistence will not be in vain, for you will reap a harvest at the proper time.

REFLECTION

Read Nehemiah 4:6 and James 1:12.

- How do these verses encourage you to remain steadfast during burdensome times?
- Write about a personal experience when perseverance through a trial led to a significant spiritual reward or personal growth.
- Use this journal to keep track of the small wins during your journey with cancer. Don't forget to write about the wins you've already experienced. They will remind you how God is present and leading you through difficult times.

PART SEVEN

Trusting in God's Timing

*I waited patiently for the Lord to help me,
and he turned to me and heard my cry.*

PSALM 40:1 NLT

DAY 31

A Time for Patience

I enjoy wearing hats. From baseball hats to Scally caps, I have a nice collection and seldom leave the house without one. Hats have been my friends and constant companions. I've also worn different "hats" throughout my professional career. Little did I know that in June 2019, a different hat would be placed upon my head when we received the diagnosis of stage 4 cancer; this new hat was emblazoned with the words *cancer patient*. God's grace and mercy guided me through the fear of diagnosis. The new hat grew tighter during treatments and tests, but God is faithful. My wife and I are still waiting patiently for His faithful direction.

In the New Testament, James 5:7-11 uses the ancient Greek word *makrothumeō* to describe patience. It means "to be slow towards, be long-enduring; to exercise patience, be long-suffering with patient expectation."[1] This kind of patience is not about remaining serene at a long red light; it better describes the enduring stamina required to finish a challenging 10K run. Pastor Charles Stanley wrote,

> It isn't easy to wait patiently before the Lord until you are sure that you have the fullness of His message to you. But how much more satisfying are the results when you know that you have heard God's entire message![2]

Chemotherapy and cancer treatments are not swift processes. Since mid-2019, I've been under continuous and various treatments. Patience becomes essential as we endure numerous sessions, scans, tests, and recovery periods, understanding that healing is a gradual journey.

Remember, God knows our sufferings. Pastor R. Kent Hughes beautifully wrote,

> God does not expect stoic perseverance in the midst of trials. He knows we are clay. He understands tears. He accepts our questions. But he does demand that we recognize our finiteness and acknowledge there are processes at work beyond our comprehension. A plan far bigger than us is moving toward completion. And God

demands that we, like Job, hold on to our faith and hope in God.[3]

Psalm 27:14 says, "Wait for the Lord; be strong and take heart and wait for the Lord" (NIV). Patience during illness and treatment reflects a profound trust in God's plan and timing. Waiting is not passive. We may not be doing anything physically, but spiritually, we are believing something unique will happen at any moment that only God can bring to pass.

A CLOSING THOUGHT

The emotional toll of cancer and its treatments can be overwhelming. Patience, that active endurance, allows individuals to navigate the roller coaster of emotions, offering the necessary margin to process fear, anger, anxiety, bitterness, and sadness.

REFLECTION

Read Habakkuk 2:3 and Romans 8:25.

- How do these verses shape your understanding of God's timing and patience in your own life?

- How can you cultivate patience, endurance, and hope in your daily life, especially during times of uncertainty and waiting?

DAY 32

Faith Is Waiting for God's Timing Without Knowing "When"

It can be challenging to wait for something interminably. Patience is a virtue and a fruit of the Spirit, but patience is difficult, especially when waiting for God's timing. The stories of Noah, Abraham, and Moses show us how hard it can be to trust in God's plan without knowing when it will come to fruition.

Noah faced ridicule and doubt as he spent an approximated 120 years waiting for God's promised flood (Genesis 6:14-22). Despite the challenges, he trusted in God's timing, and his patience was eventually rewarded (Genesis 8:1-5).

Abraham and Sarah also faced a long wait for God to fulfill the promise of children that He made to Abraham in Genesis 12:2-3. They remained childless for many years, but through this wait, their faith was strengthened. This teaches us that God's promises often require seasons of waiting that build our trust and dependence on Him (Genesis 21:1-7).

Moses, too, experienced a long period of waiting. He led the children of Israel out of bondage at the age of 80. They wandered in the wilderness for 40 years, seemingly without purpose. He was 120 when the promised land was in sight. His story underscores that God's timing is perfect, even when it seems delayed (Exodus 2:1-5; 3:1-10). His plans are beyond our understanding.

Cancer patients are in a season of waiting. Holding on to our faith and trusting God's promises and timing is essential, even when the fulfillment of those promises seems impossible. Waiting on God is difficult, but patience testifies to our faith. We can trust that in His perfect timing, He will bring His promises to fruition.

The lives of Noah, Abraham, and Moses teach us that faith involves waiting for God's "when." This waiting is not passive, but active trust and obedience. In faith, we believe God's plans are perfect and His timing is impeccable.

A CLOSING THOUGHT

If you are in a season of waiting, take heart. Like Noah, operate in faith, even when it seems foolish. Like Abraham, hold on to God's promises even when fulfillment seems impossible. Like Moses, trust and have faith that God is preparing you for His purposes, even while you are in the wilderness.

REFLECTION

Read Psalm 5:3, Psalm 33:20, and Isaiah 40:31.

- Reflect on the phrase in Psalm 33:20: "We wait in hope for the Lord" (NIV). How can you actively wait with hope during challenging times?

- In what ways does waiting for God strengthen your faith?

- Isaiah 40:31 promises renewed strength to "those who hope in the Lord" (NIV). What are practical steps we can take to place our hope in the Lord daily and trust Him in the waiting?

DAY 33

Strength from Enduring Patience

I've found that through the up-and-down journey of my cancer and treatments, the challenges often seem insurmountable. The experience has tested not only my physical body, but also my attitude and spirit. In times of trial, I find comfort in the timeless teachings of the Bible, which bring me a profound sense of inner peace. I found one such source of wisdom from the book of Job. In this fascinating and often surprising book, God offers us a beacon of hope as we navigate the various stages of illness.

The story of Job—a righteous man who faced unimaginable suffering—provides a blueprint for enduring hardships with persistent patience and unwavering faith. Pastor David Jeremiah wrote concerning God's sovereignty and Job, "Though he was assailed with greater calamities than most of us will ever face, he never rebelled against God. He grew impatient at times, and he even had to have his perspective about God corrected. But during his trials, a prayer of surrender was frequently on his lips."[1] Job's steadfastness serves as an inspiration for cancer patients grappling with the uncertainties and difficulties of the disease.

Job's story begins with him as a man who, despite being righteous, faces a series of tragic events, including the loss of his family, health, and possessions. Job's response, however, is a testament to understanding the sovereignty of God. During his suffering, Job declares, "Naked I came from my mother's womb, and naked shall I return there. The LORD gave, and the LORD has taken away; blessed be the name of the LORD" (Job 1:21). This profound acknowledgment of God's authority and control over all aspects of life lays the foundation for patience in the face of adversity.

For cancer patients, the path to healing is often long and arduous. It requires endurance, both physically and emotionally. Embracing the virtue of patience becomes a transformative aspect of this journey. Recognizing that healing is a process and not an instant resolution grants us a better understanding of God's purpose.

In times of uncertainty during cancer treatment, patients may also experience the silence of withheld answers. However, Job's example shows there is comfort and strength in seeking God's presence even when immediate explanations are not available.

Patience is not passive acceptance but an active practice of resilience. Job did not merely endure; he continued to trust and hope in God's faithfulness. We can draw inspiration from this resilience, understanding that each day is a step forward, an exercise in inner strength and determination.

The book of Job offers a guiding light, illuminating the path of patience, endurance, and faith. As cancer patients, we can find comfort in understanding that our journey is part of a grander narrative, and through patience, we can emerge more robust, resilient, and with a deeper connection to the Lord.

A CLOSING THOUGHT

In patience, there is strength; in endurance, there is growth; and in faith, there is healing. Embrace each moment, drawing inspiration from the timeless lessons of Job, and let your story become a beacon of hope for others.

REFLECTION

Read Job 23:10-14.

- How does trusting in God's unchangeable nature and sovereign plans help you navigate uncertainties and trials with patience?

- Can you think of a difficult time when patience brought peace or clarity? Explain.

DAY 34

God's Timing and Patient Endurance

When I was in the ninth grade, our teacher assigned us to write an occupational notebook: a term paper that looked ahead to how we thought we'd be working and living out our dream future. I still have mine. My notebook shows that at age 14, I thought I would attend USC, become a successful attorney, drive a Jaguar XK-E, and live not in Southern California, but in a penthouse apartment in Phoenix, Arizona, unmarried.

Why Phoenix? When I was 11 years of age, the US government contracted my father to appraise specific areas of land, which contained parts of the Apache reservation. We were headquartered for several weeks in Show Low, Arizona, and spent many days in and around Phoenix. As a child, I fell in love with the city and what I thought it offered.

I never lived in Phoenix. I married (54 years ago and counting) and didn't become a lawyer or own an XK-E. Our family lived in San Bernardino, California (our hometown); San Juan Capistrano, California; Ann Arbor, Michigan; Arroyo Grande, California; Franklin, Tennessee; and Kingston Springs, Tennessee. We needed to patiently learn to live where God put us.

How does all this relate to my battle with cancer? Well, like my family amid our moves, we're each learning to have patience with where God has put us—not in new cities, but in a chemotherapy room, hospital, and oncology office. Adapting to new cultures can be difficult, but we must adapt if we hope to rise above grumbling and despair. For example, a kid from sunny California may struggle when suddenly relocated to Ann Arbor, Michigan, where there is an abundance of ice, snow, and cold (but no ocean).

Jeremiah 29 is a chapter in the Bible that deals with this idea of living fully where you are. In a letter to the Babylonian exiles, the Lord said,

> Build houses and dwell in them; plant gardens and eat their fruit. Take wives and beget sons and daughters; and take wives for your sons and give your daughters to husbands, so that they may bear sons and

daughters—that you may be increased there, and not diminished. And seek the peace of the city where I have caused you to be carried away captive, and pray to the Lord for it; for in its peace you will have peace (Jeremiah 29:5-7).

Do you want peace? Be patient, trust God and His timing, and try to flourish where the Lord has put you. Build houses, have a family, pray, and peacefully follow where He guides you. God wanted Israel to do good in their Babylonian communities and bless their neighbors. After all, God had led them to Babylon—so He wanted them to be a blessing where He'd put them.

Accepting where God has placed me has implications for my cancer experience. I find myself in various rooms with nurses, technicians, doctors, and patients, many of whom are in far more pain than I. Should I complain? Should I be bitter? No. I must live and have peace where God has put me. I must try to be as kind and generous as I can be. Some patients and workers need to see *chesed*, the Hebrew word often translated as loving-kindness. I believe God has put Pam and me in those places for a reason.

We can choose to fight our circumstances, or we can seek patience and peace when we find ourselves in a difficult place. Then we can try, with God's help, to encourage others around us.

A CLOSING THOUGHT

Bishop William Bernard Ullathorne said,

> By the virtue of patient endurance, the gift of God, we possess the government of our souls, and keep our peaceful recollection in the face of all our adversaries…the daily exercise of patience and endurance we are prepared for the hour of trial, which for us is the hour of combat.[1]

REFLECTION

Read Luke 21:19 and Hebrews 10:36.

- In your journal, list ways you can stand firm in the place God has placed you.
- Pause and pray for God to help you stand firm in patient endurance.

DAY 35

Trusting in God's Timing

Waiting is often one of the most challenging aspects of life, especially for those battling cancer. The journey involves waiting for test results, treatment plans, and the effects of medication. In these waiting periods, we face crucial choices with consequences that can impact our spiritual, emotional, and physical well-being.

In our impatience, we may be tempted to manipulate circumstances to achieve our desired results. This attitude might lead us to pursue alternative treatments without proper guidance or make hasty decisions about care or life in general. Acting outside of God's will often result in consequences that can hinder our healing process and spiritual growth. Proverbs 14:12 warns, "There is a way that seems right to a man, but its end is the way of death." Impatience and resistance to God's path can lead us into spiritual emptiness and unnecessary suffering.

Another temptation we face is quitting and walking

away. The emotional and physical toll of cancer can be overwhelming, leading some to consider giving up on treatments or losing faith in God's plan and purpose. Yet abandoning the course means missing out on God's best for us. The book of Hebrews points out how Abraham waited for God: "After he had patiently endured, he obtained the promise" (Hebrews 6:15). The valuable things in life often require a long and patient wait.

The most rewarding choice is to wait and watch God work. Waiting requires trusting in His perfect timing and knowing His will is best for our lives. Psalm 25:5 reminds us, "Lead me in Your truth and teach me, for You are the God of my salvation; on You I wait all the day." We gain new strength and perspective when we wait on God, and with Him, we can endure the journey with hope and resilience.

While our desires may push us toward immediate gratification, God calls us to respond to His plans and timing for our lives. He promises to direct our paths if we trust in Him. Psalm 16:11 advises, "You will show me the path of life; in Your presence is fullness of joy; at Your right hand are pleasures forevermore." We will find God's joy when we exchange our plans and timing for His perfect will.

A CLOSING THOUGHT

As cancer patients, the waiting periods are inevitable and often complicated. However, our choices during these times can lead us closer to God's best for our lives. By resisting the urge to manipulate our circumstances and instead choosing to wait on God, we allow Him to work in and through us in powerful ways. Trust in His timing.

REFLECTION

Read Psalms 27:14 and 37:34.

- How can you actively "take heart" and find strength during waiting periods?
- In your journal, note some practical steps you can take to remain hopeful and patient while trusting God's timing and promises.

PART EIGHT

Welcoming Endurance and Hope

Rejoice in our confident hope. Be patient in trouble, and keep on praying.

ROMANS 12:12 NLT

DAY 36

Beyond the Thorn

Unexpected injuries and disease bring a host of emotions—fear, loss, and insecurity among them. A whole array of emotions hit Pam and me as we sat in the doctor's office and heard the initial cancer diagnosis. As we walk this journey, we have a choice: We can mourn our situation, or we can, like the apostle Paul, pray hard, persevere, and stay on the course God has for us with endurance and hope.

In 2 Corinthians 12:7, Paul wrote about his "thorn in the flesh." Many scholars guess what his thorn might have been, but Paul never specified his exact ailment. He prayed three times for this "thorn" to disappear, but it didn't. Instead, God told him, "My grace is sufficient for you, for My strength is made perfect in weakness." To which Paul responded: "Therefore, most gladly I will rather boast in my infirmities, that the power of Christ may rest upon me" (2 Corinthians 12:9).

God's strength is perfected in weakness. Paul reveals that we Christians have a race to run, and he urges Christians to run with hope, discipline, and determination (1 Corinthians 9:24-27). He played the game hard. He looked to God instead of his thorn, which he saw as a gift from God to mature him and give him purpose—his calling.

In Galatians 4:13, Paul writes to the people of Galatia about another time he needed God's strength to be made perfect in his weakness. He suffered a "physical infirmity" yet never allowed his infirmity to get in the way of delivering God's message and fulfilling God's plan and purposes. His example compels us to face our adversities—whether cancer, injury, or any other trial—head-on, trusting that God's grace is sufficient.

Dealing with cancer and cancer treatments isn't easy. I've found myself allowing my emotions to get the best of me. I've succumbed to fear, anger, and that question of "why me"? But even at my lowest points, I remember Paul. He ran the race with hope despite his thorn. While Satan wanted to destroy Paul's endurance and ministry, God planned to develop Paul's faith through hardship. Paul responded as we should: by knowing that God's strength is perfected in our weakness. He will give us strength when we need it. He will give us hope. Bible commentator William Barclay wrote,

Note that it never struck [Paul] to turn back. Even when his body was aching, Paul never stopped driving himself forward as an adventurer for Christ.[1]

A CLOSING THOUGHT

In 2 Corinthians 12:9, Paul describes how God's grace is sufficient for us, for His power is made perfect in our weakness. This assurance gives us hope, strength, and endurance—the fruits of knowing God's grace sustains us and turns our weaknesses into displays of His strength.

REFLECTION

Read Job 22:27-29 and Psalm 43:5.

- In what ways can these verses lift your spirits when you're feeling hopeless or overwhelmed?
- In your journal, list some practical steps you can take to refocus your mind on hope and praise, even in difficult circumstances.

DAY 37

Choosing Hope When Everything Looks Hopeless

Hope is a choice—not wishful thinking. Hope is a confident expectation that something good is going to happen. It's a choice we make as we deal with cancer and all the emotions and thoughts that come with the disease and treatment. Hope is significant because choosing it has many benefits. Harvard Medical School assistant professor Adam P. Stern, MD, wrote:

> Hope can be a particularly powerful protector against the dread of a chronic or life-threatening illness. It needn't center on a cure to be useful, though those aspirations are enticing. Rather, a person's hope—even when facing an illness…can be aimed at finding joy or comfort.[1]

The Bible offers profound wisdom and encouragement, reminding us that hope is not just an emotion but a deliberate choice. During the darkest trials, we can choose to hold onto hope, knowing God's promises and presence are steadfast.

The Bible repeatedly calls us to hope in God, even when circumstances seem dire. Here is a powerful example in Psalm 42:11: "Why are you cast down, O my soul? And why are you disquieted within me? Hope in God; for I shall yet praise Him, the help of my countenance and my God." The psalmist is determined to hope in the Lord. He decides to redirect his focus from overwhelming circumstances toward faith and confidence in God.

Choosing hope means deliberately placing our trust in God's Word and His promises, despite what our circumstances may suggest. The apostle Paul offers a beautiful prayer:

> I pray that God, the source of hope, will *fill you completely with joy and peace* because you trust in him. Then you will *overflow with confident hope* through the power of the Holy Spirit (Romans 15:13 NLT, emphasis mine).

He is the God of our *hope*. Trust in Him to overcome hopelessness. Pastor Rick Warren said,

Hope is the anchor of the soul. [It is a] thing that I can count on, so that no matter what happens, I know that life is not hopeless.[2]

A CLOSING THOUGHT

Remember, hope is a choice rooted in God's unwavering love and faithfulness. Let us cling to this hope, knowing He is turning our moments of despair into opportunities for us to realize His grace, power, and glory.

REFLECTION

Read Psalms 33:22 and 73:26.

- In your journal, list ways to practice putting your hope in God amid emotional distress or discouragement.
- What specific actions or habits can help you focus on praising God in difficult times?

DAY 38

The Power of Hope in God's Plan

Often cancer can feel insurmountable. It can enclose me in shadows of doubt and despair. Sometimes I feel as if I'm on an elevator, riding up and down depending on my current emotions, all resulting from the disease. In the down moments, hope becomes a lifeline. As we have seen before in an earlier devotional, Romans 8:28 offers a profound reassurance: "We know that all things work together for good to those who love God, to those who are the called according to His purpose." This verse reminds me that my circumstances, no matter how dire, are under God's sovereign control and are part of His plan for my good.

Hope is not just a fleeting feeling, but a confident expectation rooted in the character and promises of God. While we can know beyond a doubt that God's sovereignty ultimately controls our lives and emotions, we don't know the details of His vision. Sometimes we don't even know what to pray for. To keep our feelings and ruminations from running amok, we need to focus on what we know: His Word, our prayers, and what He has done for us in the past.

Also, Romans 8:28 assures us that God is actively working in "all things" for the good of those who love Him. This phrase means He takes what happens and weaves it into a plan for my good and His glory. He turns every moment of a cancer journey—every treatment, every setback, and every victory—into ultimate blessings according to His purpose. Believing in this promise requires hope. This hope enables us to trust that God is in control. We need to join Paul in expressing faith in the goodness of God's purpose for us even when our situations seem hopeless.

Hope in God's promises strengthens us and assures us He is working on our situation. The Bible has many examples of God intervening in seemingly impossible situations. We must hold onto the hope that God can and will work similarly in our lives, transforming our circumstances according to His perfect will.

Philippians 4:19 reassures us, "My God will meet all your needs according to the riches of his glory in Christ Jesus" (NIV). This promise, coupled with the assurance of Romans 8:28, provides a strong foundation for our hope. We can trust that God not only understands our needs but also is fully capable of meeting them. This truth can fill us with confident hope, strength, comfort, and peace as we navigate the cancer journey.

A CLOSING THOUGHT

We can experience a profound freedom from worry because God is sovereign and working all things to our benefit. He assures us that He will make good of our circumstances, holding everything in His capable hands.

REFLECTION

Read Psalms 103:13 and 135:6.

- How does recognizing God's sovereignty over all creation provide comfort and assurance in times of uncertainty or struggle?

- What specific instance do you recall wherein trusting God's sovereignty brought you peace?

- How can remembering this instance help you as you face new and seemingly hopeless situations?

DAY 39

Embracing Hope over Negativity

Biblical hope is a favorable and confident expectation. Hope is a positive attitude—not a thought or a feeling, but a stance focused solely on God's promises. We find a profound truth in Psalm 38:15: "For in You, O Lord, I hope; You will hear, O Lord my God." This verse summarizes a powerful principle: We have the choice to remain hopeful, even when circumstances seem bleak.

The hopeful person refuses to be negative. While fully recognizing and dealing with life's circumstances, they maintain a hopeful outlook in thought, attitude, and conversation. This principle is crucial for cancer patients. Acknowledging the reality of our situations does not mean succumbing to despair. Instead, we can choose to speak words of faith and hope, aligning our hearts with God's promises because, as the psalmist declared, He hears!

Our speech reflects our faith; therefore, we cannot say we trust God to move in our lives while simultaneously talking and acting as if nothing good can happen. James 3:10 reminds us, "Blessing and cursing come pouring out of the same mouth. Surely, my brothers and sisters, this is not right!" (NLT). Our words have power; they can either build up our faith or tear it down. By consistently speaking hope and having a positive attitude, we reinforce our trust in God's ability to work out all things, even through the most challenging circumstances (Romans 8:28).

A negative mindset goes against the biblical teachings that encourage believers to focus on thoughts that are true, honorable, just, pure, lovely, commendable, and worthy of praise (Philippians 4:8). When we face obstacles, it's easy to let our hope erode—leading us to speak and think negatively and set aside what Philippians 4:8 teaches us. This negativity can become a destructive cycle, as it seeps into our own pessimistic viewpoint, attracts others who share our bleak outlook, and amplifies our despair. As we spiral downward, we distance ourselves from God's promises, which thrive in an internal atmosphere of faith in Him and His Word. As believers, we must consciously choose to reject negativity, hold fast to hope, and speak words of faith, aligning ourselves with the truth of God's unwavering promises.

A CLOSING THOUGHT

By remaining hopeful, we align ourselves with God's promises and invite His peace and strength into our lives. Remember, hope is not a fleeting feeling, but a steadfast decision to trust in the God who never fails. As you work through this challenging journey, may you be filled with unwavering hope, knowing that the Lord your God is with you and will answer you.

REFLECTION

Read Zechariah 9:12 and 1 Peter 1:3.

- In your opinion, what does "prisoners of hope" mean in Zechariah 9:12?
- How can this concept transform your perspective on difficult circumstances?
- In your journal, write about a time when clinging to hope led to restoration in your life.

DAY 40

God's Anchor of Hope

In Genesis 15, we find Abram (before God changed his name to Abraham) in doubt. God has already promised Abram that He will make him into "a great nation" (12:2), and He has led Abram to land He says He will give to Abram's descendants (12:7; 13:15). Abram has followed the instructions God has given him (12:4) and seemingly remained confident in God's promises—yet he is still without a child. Here we see him breaking down, but God tells him: "Do not be afraid, Abram. I am your shield, your exceedingly great reward" (15:1).

Abram responds with despair:

> O Sovereign Lord, what good are all your blessings when I don't even have a son?… You have given me no descendants of my own, so one of my servants will be my heir (Genesis 15:2-3 NLT).

In this dark moment of Abram's discouragement, God reassures Abram of His promises:

> "No, your servant will not be your heir, for you will have a son of your own who will be your heir." Then the Lord took Abram outside and said to him, "Look up into the sky and count the stars if you can. That's how many descendants you will have!" (verse 4 NLT).

At these words, we see Abram meet God's reassurance with a heart of trust and confidence: "Abram believed the Lord, and the Lord counted him as righteous because of his faith" (verse 6 NLT).

Having hope in God's message became an anchor for Abram.

When you drop an anchor, your boat is secured and can only move so far. Despite cancer and all that comes with the disease, we can be anchored steadfastly in God's hope. When our anchor is down, we don't drift; we stay connected to God. He keeps us secure and stable. When we are confident in God's promises to be "close to the brokenhearted" and rescue "those whose spirits are crushed" (Psalm 34:18 NLT), we are anchored in calm waters and protected from drifting into the stormy sea of fear, despair, anger, bitterness, and self-pity.

Later in Genesis, we see Joseph, the son of Jacob, facing many opportunities to pull up his anchor of hope and drift away into despair. Yet despite being sold into slavery and wrongfully imprisoned, his faith in God remains intact. The Lord stays with him when he is a slave in Potiphar's house and when he is imprisoned under false charges (Genesis 39), and Joseph's faithfulness is so clear that he becomes known to Pharaoh as a "man so obviously filled with the spirit of God" (Genesis 41:38 NLT).

King David is another person anchored by his hope in God. When David confronts Goliath, the giant warrior, he never pulls up this anchor. Despite the protests of onlookers who see his battle as impossible, David proclaims, "The LORD, who delivered me from the paw of the lion and from the paw of the bear, He will deliver me from the hand of this Philistine" (1 Samuel 17:37). In the face of tremendous and frightening struggles, Joseph and David offer examples of how to remain anchored to the One who gives us strength, courage, and purpose.

A lack of hope weakens us. Hopelessness can result in depression and anxiety, undermining any positive efforts and trivializing any small victories. Hope is the strength that carries us through today and all tomorrows, and we are fueled by trusting the Lord. Hope wakes us up each morning with gratitude for the blessings He's given. Hope is powerful, keeping us securely anchored to God's Word, ways, will, and promises.

A CLOSING THOUGHT

Abram needed assurance, and God made a promise to him. Over time, Abram held onto the promise with incredible faith and hope. Similarly, we can be prisoners of hope as we lean on and trust God in all things. He is working in our lives for our ultimate good.

REFLECTION

Read Psalm 146:5-6, Isaiah 12:2, and Jeremiah 17:7. Journal your responses to these questions:

- What does it mean to place your complete confidence and hope in the Lord, especially amid life's challenges and uncertainties?
- List ways you can build and maintain this trust actively and maintain hope in God.

Closing Thoughts
Moving Forward

I want to provide some final thoughts as I finish writing this devotional. As I've traveled this challenging cancer journey, my life verse has served to strengthen and encourage me. So, in closing, let's examine Proverbs 3:5-7:

> Trust in the Lord with all your heart, and lean not on your understanding; in all your ways acknowledge Him, and He shall direct your paths. Do not be wise in your own eyes; fear the Lord and depart from evil.

Or as *The Message* translates it:

> Trust God from the bottom of your heart; don't try to figure out everything on your

> own. Listen for God's voice in everything you do, everywhere you go; he's the one who will keep you on track. Don't assume that you know it all. Run to God! Run from evil!

This powerful verse captures many key principles we've discussed: grace, navigating the unknown, vulnerability, joy, purpose, small victories, God's timing, and hope.

Trust the Lord. To trust God means embracing vulnerability and acknowledging your need for His strength and guidance. It's about letting go of the need to understand everything and, instead, leaning and relying on Him, trusting in His infinite wisdom and loving care. We can't overcome the challenges through our limited wisdom; instead, we must trust God. Ultimately, we need to be satisfied with knowing the One who knows.

With all your heart. Nothing short of total commitment to God is required. Deuteronomy 6:5 tells us, "You shall love the Lord your God with all your heart, with all your soul, and with all your strength." The word *all* means being fully engaged. Pastor Charles Stanley, commenting on Deuteronomy 6:5, wrote: "We are to love Him with all of the heart, the seat of the emotions; with all of the soul, the core of personality; with all of our strength, all that is within us; with all of our might—consumed with Him."[1]

In all your ways acknowledge Him. I've learned I am not smart enough to run my life. The Hebrew word translated as "acknowledge" is *yada*, also commonly translated as "to know." Scripture frequently uses this word to denote a covenant relationship between two people. Tim Hegg, biblical scholar and overseer at Beit Hallel in Tacoma, Washington, wrote, "In the Ancient Near East, a covenant between two people or between a King and his people was considered to be a relationship that could not be broken and that if it were to be broken, there would result severe consequences (the curses of the covenant)."[2] I can choose to do things on my own, or I can know and deeply connect with God and His ways.

And He shall direct your paths. As we trust in God, know Him deeply, and submit to His ways, He promises to set our course. This promise doesn't mean life will be easy, but He will guide us, provide for us, and bring us to the other side. His plans are always for our good, and His love for us is unwavering. According to one study Bible, "[The Hebrew word] *Yashar*, lit. 'to make smooth, straight, right,' includes the idea of removing obstacles that are in the way. God will straighten the stressful paths. He does not say when or how; He just promises that He will."[3]

I encourage you to hold onto these truths and let them be your anchor through the challenges of cancer. Trust in the Lord with all your heart. He is with you every step of the way, making your paths straight and leading you toward His perfect purpose and plan for your life.

Afterword

On Tuesday, October 1, 2024, with his family by his side, their voices united with a choir of angels, Wayne was welcomed to his eternal home. Now completely healed and fully redeemed—halleluiah!—he is with the King. "As for me, I shall behold your face in righteousness; when I awake, I shall be satisfied with your likeness" (Psalm 17:15 ESV).

Born in San Bernardino, California, the son of Ray and Catherine Hastings, Wayne was an all-around athlete and Big Man on Campus. He met the love of his life, Pamela Lorraine, in biology lab when they were seniors. It was love at first sight. On June 6, 1970, Wayne and Pam vowed to be best friends and partners for life. June 2024 marked 54 years of walking hand in hand. Their love story became intertwined with their faith story. Together, Wayne and Pam received the gift of salvation through their Lord and Savior, Jesus Christ. The Lord blessed them with two children, Jennifer Rebecca and Zachary Todd. Wayne and Pam's family grew to include Jennifer's husband, Deron, and Zachary's wife, Anna. Wayne was Pop-Pop to Becky, Abby, Claire, and Todd.

Wayne's accomplished career in Christian publishing included various roles: author, editor, marketer, and mentor. His goal was to place life-changing materials in the hands of others in order to equip and encourage them in their walk with Christ. Wayne was a music lover, a skilled guitarist, and a lifelong Los Angeles Dodgers fan. Above all, Wayne is a child of God. He embraced Jesus Christ as his personal Lord and Savior. In this life, God's presence filled him with wisdom and strength. He never wavered in his belief of God's Word and promises. He lived by the assurance that every prayer was heard.

On the evening of August 27, my dad sent me a text asking me how I was. Earlier that day we had received the news that treatment would need to end. I replied, "Well, the blessing of today is that you gave me the gift of our eternal Father. I can be heartbroken and yet know that you and I share a faith that will not only see us through, but will also hold us for eternity. We've got this because He's got us."

With a fighting determination and singular focus, Wayne completed this manuscript just days before he became too ill to write. His commitment to the writing of these words of encouragement and truth came from a passion to offer hope, guidance, and comfort. We are inspired by his example and humbled by the privilege of seeing his words published.

Our family is truly thankful for the generous prayers and blessed encouragement from so many during these past months. Faithful friends continue to uplift and sustain us as we navigate this path of grief. We rejoice though we are heartbroken. We cherish memories while taking many new and unfamiliar steps. We remind each other that he loved us. We await the day when we will see him again.

We gratefully offer his words in closing.

With love, grace, and unwavering hope,
Jennifer Cook, on behalf of the Hastings family

Notes

DAY 1: GRACE THROUGH FAITH

1. *The Lexham Bible Dictionary* (Bellingham, WA: Lexham Press, 2016), under "grace."
2. David Platt, Jim Shaddix, and Matt Mason, *Exalting Jesus in Psalms 51-100* (Nashville, TN: Holman Reference, 2020), 326.

DAY 2: ECHOES OF GRACE

1. David Platt, Jim Shaddix, and Matt Mason, *Exalting Jesus in Psalms 51-100* (Nashville, TN: Holman Reference, 2020), 280.

DAY 3: SAVED BY GRACE

1. Charles H. Spurgeon, *The Treasury of David, Volume 2: Psalms 27–57*, Logos Bible Software Edition.

DAY 4: LIFE CHANGES QUICKLY

1. *Collins COBUILD Idioms Dictionary*, "turn on a dime," accessed June 11, 2024, https://idioms.thefreedictionary.com/turn+on+a+dime.
2. James Montgomery Boice, *Psalms 42–106: An Expositional Commentary* (Grand Rapids, MI: Baker Books, 2005), 392.
3. "Wesley's Last Hours" Christian Classics Ethereal Library, accessed January 31, 2025, at https://www.ccel.org/ccel/wesley/journal.vi.xxi.html

DAY 6: NAVIGATING THE UNKNOWN

1. Steve Turner, *Turn, Turn, Turn: Popular Songs Inspired by the Bible* (Nashville, TN: Worthy Books in association with Museum of the Bible, 2018), 78.
2. Charles R. Swindoll and Roy B. Zuck, *Understanding Christian Theology* (Nashville, TN: Thomas Nelson, 2003), 222.
3. Warren W. Wiersbe, *Be Satisfied*, "Be" Commentary Series (Wheaton, IL: Victor Books, 1996), 45.

DAY 7: LIFE'S SIDE EFFECTS

1. Charles Stanley, *Eternal Security: Can You Be Sure?* (Nashville, TN: Thomas Nelson, 1990), 6-7.

DAY 8: BALANCING ACT

1. John Stott with Dale and Sandy Larsen, *Reading Galatians with John Stott: 9 Weeks for Individuals or Groups* (Downers Grove, IL: IVP Connect, 2017), 108.

DAY 9: ANCHORING HOPE

1. John Piper, *Sermons from John Piper (1990–1999)* (Minneapolis, MN: Desiring God, 2007).
2. Arthur Walkington Pink, *Gleanings from Paul Studies in the Prayers of the Apostle* (Bellingham, WA: Logos Bible Software, 2005), 39.

DAY 11: EMBRACING DIVINE VULNERABILITY

1. Colin G. Kruse, *2 Corinthians: An Introduction and Commentary*, vol. 8, Tyndale New Testament Commentaries (Downers Grove, IL: InterVarsity Press, 1987), 200.

DAY 12: BREAKING THE CHAINS OF EMOTIONAL RESTRAINT

1. *The Complete Word Study Dictionary*, ed. Spiros Zodhiates (Chattanooga, TN: AMG International, Inc., 1992), e-Sword X electronic edition, under "dakka."
2. Warren W. Wiersbe, *With the Word: The Chapter-by-Chapter Bible Handbook* (Nashville, TN: Thomas Nelson, 1991), under "Psalm 34."
3. *Brown-Driver-Briggs Hebrew Definitions*, published 1906, public domain. e-Sword X electronic edition.

DAY 13: LEARNING FROM A KING

1. Menachem Posner, "15 Life-lessons from King David," Chabad.org, accessed June 22, 2024, https://www.chabad.org/library/article_cdo/aid/4114664/jewish/15-Life-Lessons-From-King-David.htm.

DAY 14: FINDING HOPE THROUGH LAMENT

1. *Collins Dictionary*, "lament," accessed June 22, 2024, https://www.collinsdictionary.com/dictionary/english/lament.

DAY 15: FLOURISHING IN VULNERABILITY

1. William Barclay, *The Letter to the Hebrews*, The New Daily Study Bible (Louisville, KY; Westminster John Knox Press, 2002), 52.

DAY 16: HARMONIZING HOPE

1. Roger Ellsworth, *Opening up Philippians*, Opening Up Commentary (Leominster: Day One Publications, 2004), 83.
2. James MacDonald, "Outrageous Counting," Harvest Compassion Center, December 20, 2016, https://harvestcompassioncenter.org/outrageous-counting/.

DAY 17: EMBRACING JOYFUL GRATITUDE

1. Talmud, Berachot: 7b, trans. Adin Even-Israel (Steinsaltz), Chabad.org, accessed January 10, 2024, https://www.chabad.org/torah-texts/5299487/The-Talmud/Berachot/Chapter-1/7b.
2. Jacob's sons came from four women: Leah, Rachel, Bilha, and Zilpah. Leah had expected that each woman would have three sons.
3. Rabbi Shai Held, *The Heart of Torah: Essays on the Weekly Torah Portion: Genesis, Exodus, Leviticus, Numbers, and Deuteronomy*, vol. 1 (Philadelphia, PA: The Jewish Publication Society, 2017), 63.

DAY 18: FINDING SHALOM IN THE STILLNESS

1. Doug Hershey, "The True Meaning of Shalom," FIRM Israel, January 3, 2020, https://firmisrael.org/learn/the-meaning-of-shalom/.
2. "Lexicon: Strong's H1826—*dāmam*," accessed June 25, 2024, https://www.blueletterbible.org/lexicon/h1826/kjv/wlc/0-1/.

DAY 19: TWO OF US

1. Paul McCartney, *The Lyrics: 1956 to Present* (New York: Liveright Publishing, 2021), 497.

DAY 20: FINDING JOY DESPITE ALL THAT'S BAD

1. Rick Warren, "What Is the Secret to Joy in Life? Ask Pastor Rick," from the sermon, "You Are Called to Bless," posted August 31, 2015. https://www.youtube.com/watch?v=CV0iSF6_8Dk.

2. "Cancer," World Health Organization, February 3, 2020, https://www.who.int/news-room/fact-sheets/detail/cancer.

DAY 21: FINDING PURPOSE THROUGH DIFFICULTY

1. "Quote Origin: Two Most Important Days in Your Life: The Day You Were Born and the Day You Discover Why," Quote Investigator, June 22, 2016, https://quoteinvestigator.com/2016/06/22/why/.
2. Kathie Lee Gifford and Rabbi Jason Sobel, *The God of the Way* (Nashville, TN: W Publishing, 2022), 137.

DAY 22: TRUSTING GOD'S PLAN

1. Warren W. Wiersbe, *Be Decisive*, "Be" Commentary Series (Wheaton, IL: Victor Books, 1996), 124.
2. Max Lucado, *The Great House of God: A Home for Your Heart* (Dallas, TX: Word, 1997), 72.

DAY 25: LETTING YOUR LIGHT SHINE

1. Jon Courson, *Jon Courson's Application Commentary* (Nashville, TN: Thomas Nelson, 2003), 1500.

DAY 27: RESETTING EXPECTATIONS

1. Jentezen Franklin, "Celebrating the Little Victories," accessed July 3, 2024, https://jentezenfranklin.org/broadcasts/celebrating-the-little-victories.

DAY 30: PERSISTENCE AND SMALL WINS

1. Saurabh Verma, "The Miracle of Small Wins: Unleashing the Power of Incremental Progress," July 31, 2023, https://www.everymindful.com/the-miracle-of-small-wins-unleashing-the-power-of-incremental-progress.

DAY 31: A TIME FOR PATIENCE

1. Bill Mounce, "μακροθυμέω," accessed July 8, 2024, https://www.billmounce.com/greek-dictionary/makrothumeo.
2. Charles F. Stanley, *Listening to God* (Nashville, TN: Thomas Nelson, 1996), Logos Bible Software Edition.

3. R. Kent Hughes, *James: Faith That Works*, Preaching the Word Series (Wheaton, IL: Crossway Books, 1991), 239.

DAY 33: STRENGTH FROM ENDURING PATIENCE

1. David Jeremiah, *Signs of Life* (Nashville, TN: Thomas Nelson, 2007), 97.

DAY 34: GOD'S TIMING AND PATIENT ENDURANCE

1. William Bernard Ullathorne, *Christian Patience: The Strength and Discipline of the Soul* (London: Granville Mansions, 1886), 136.

DAY 36: BEYOND THE THORN

1. William Barclay, *The Acts of the Apostles*, *The New Daily Study Bible* (Louisville, KY; Westminster John Knox Press, 2003), 120.

DAY 37: CHOOSING HOPE WHEN EVERYTHING LOOKS HOPELESS

1. Adam P. Stern, "Hope: Why it matters," Harvard Health Publishing, July 16, 2021, https://www.health.harvard.edu/blog/hope-why-it-matters-202107162547.
2. Rick Warren, "Where to Find the Hope You Need—Part 1," radio broadcast, July 2, 2024, https://pastorrick.com/listen-online/where-to-find-the-hope-you-need-part-1/.

CLOSING THOUGHTS: MOVING FORWARD

1. Charles F. Stanley, *The Glorious Journey* (Nashville, TN: Thomas Nelson, 1996), Logos Bible Software.
2. Tim Hegg, "Hebrew Word Yada: As a Covenant Term in the Bible and the Ancient Near East," TorahResource, accessed July 13, 2024, https://torahresource.com/article/hebrew-word-yada/.
3. *The Woman's Study Bible* (Nashville, TN: Thomas Nelson, 1995), Proverbs 3:6.

Unless otherwise indicated, all Scripture verses are taken from the New King James Version®. Copyright © 1982 by Thomas Nelson. Used with permission. All rights reserved.

Verses marked ESV are taken from the ESV® Bible (The Holy Bible, English Standard Version®), copyright © 2001 by Crossway, a publishing ministry of Good News Publishers. Used with permission. All rights reserved. The ESV text may not be quoted in any publication made available to the public by a Creative Commons license. The ESV may not be translated in whole or in part into any other language.

Verses marked NLT are taken from the *Holy Bible*, New Living Translation, copyright © 1996, 2004, 2015 by Tyndale House Foundation. Used with permission of Tyndale House Publishers, Carol Stream, Illinois 60188. All rights reserved.

Verses marked NIV are taken from the *Holy Bible*, New International Version®, NIV®. Copyright © 1973, 1978, 1984, 2011 by Biblica, Inc.™ Used with permission of Zondervan. All rights reserved worldwide. www.zondervan.com. The "NIV" and "New International Version" are trademarks registered in the United States Patent and Trademark Office by Biblica, Inc.™

Verses marked AMP taken from the Amplified® Bible (AMP), Copyright © 2015 by The Lockman Foundation. Used with permission. www.lockman.org.

Verses marked MSG are taken from *The Message*, copyright © 1993, 2002, 2018 by Eugene H. Peterson. Used with permission of NavPress. All rights reserved. Represented by Tyndale House Publishers, Inc.

Verses marked AMPC are taken from the Amplified® Bible (AMPC), Copyright © 1954, 1958, 1962, 1964, 1965, 1987 by The Lockman Foundation Used with permission. lockman.org

Verses marked TLV are taken from the Holy Scriptures, Tree of Life Version, copyright © 2014, 2016 by the Tree of Life Bible Society. Used with permission of the Tree of Life Bible Society.